D0886634

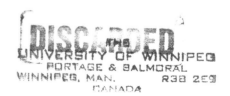

The Aged in the Community

Dwight Frankfather

The Praeger Special Studies program—
utilizing the most modern and efficient book
production techniques and a selective
worldwide distribution network—makes
available to the academic, government, and
business communities significant, timely
research in U.S. and international eco
nomic, social, and political development

The Aged in the Community
Managing Senility and Deviance

Praeger Publishers   New York   London

Library of Congress Cataloging in Publication Data

Frankfather, Dwight, 1946-
    The aged in the community

    (Praeger special studies in U.S. economic, social,
and political issues)
    Bibliography: p.213
    Includes index.
    1. Geriatric psychiatry.   2. Community mental
health services.   I.   Title.
RC451.4.A5F74   362.6'12'2   77-8327
ISBN 0-03-021936-1
ISBN 0-03-021931-0 student ed.

PRAEGER PUBLISHERS
200 Park Avenue, New York, N.Y. 10017, U.S.A.

Published in the United States of America in 1977
by Praeger Publishers, Inc.

789 038 987654321

Displayed here are the experiences of a segment of older adults as they confront the urban environment. These older persons are set apart by their presumed deficiency in mental functioning. They can be seen on the streets of the inner city. In appearance they are likely to be unattractive; their behavior is likely to be bizarre. Occasionally they call attention to themselves by their public eccentricities or by seeking help in one way or another. Because so many of these persons are without family or make demands to which families cannot respond, the capacity of the organized service sector to respond is critical. The fact that services are ostensibly available only complicates the situation. Medical care, psychiatric treatment, social services and recreational facilities are present in the community. The confused elderly gravitate toward these services. But those called on to render service are not prepared to do so for this population.

There is an imbalance in the nature of services that are offered. Most readily available is sophisticated health care; yet, the problems which the confused older person presents are only incidentally medical in nature. Furthermore, the central interest of adherents to the medical model is diagnosis and treatment of conditions which they are trained to handle. Unfortunately, the confused elderly are diagnosed as beyond treatment. The characteristic reaction of medical personnel is to evade responsibility. Medication to control objectionable behavior is the principal response. Beyond that, this population is expelled from medical and psychiatric settings. Those who are thwarted by the institutions are invited to become, once again, invisible members of the urban society.

Those whose persistence or visibility demands attention are characteristically placed in nursing homes. This is not the solution that they welcome. It imposes some effective constraints on potentially unacceptable behavior, largely through surveillance and medication. While it also sustains the life of this population, it does so at substantial cost to society and to the individual who effectively loses his freedom.

As Dr. Frankfather demonstrates, the central problem of the confused elderly is the incapacity to survive on a day-to-day basis. Public programs are needed which recognize the legitimacy of their survival needs. Imaginative forms of intervention must be developed to sustain with dignity those not capable of fending for themselves. This implies a willingness on the part of service providers to do dirty work, that is, menial tasks which are basic to day-to-day existence. We must acknowledge that however essential such needs may be, they run counter to the drift toward professionalization on the part of service providers. This drift leads providers to concentrate on specialized and relatively esoteric services to the neglect of survival needs. Also implied is a willingness on the part of providers to take on a wide range of responsibilities. If the confused adult is to be relieved of the burden of negotiating a configuration of fragmented services, the tendency toward multiple categorical services must be reversed. A delicate balance must be found between respect for the autonomy of an individual and tolerance of his eccentricities, and cheerful provision of help needed to assure survival.

The study establishes the basic requirements of an adequate service configuration for this population. Specific forms of service intervention and approaches to inevitable cost issues are important subjects for professional and political debate.

Dr. Frankfather illuminates the problems in a way which pleads compellingly for greater proficiency and humanity on the part of service providers in meeting the needs of the mentally handicapped urban elderly. It is my hope that the study will stimulate both the public concern and professional attention which the problem deserves.

ACKNOWLEDGMENTS

Frank Caro and Karen Peterson deserve the recognition that one expects to find in an acknowledgment. Frank's unique skill as a social scientist and his pragmatic sensibilities were instrumental in setting a research course, and preventing at least one fatal wrong turn in the beginning. His influence has had the admirable quality of calculated self-restraint. Karen more than any other contributor influenced the appearance of the final document. Every single word, sentence, paragraph, page, and chapter was subject to her assiduous scrutiny. We argued about everything from sentence structure to the presumed logical progression of ideas to be presented. She won more arguments than she lost.

Louis Lowy, Bob Morris, and Bob Patterson read the manuscript carefully and made suggestions which influenced various sections of the paper.

CONTENTS

Chapter

Chapter

LIST OF TABLES AND FIGURE

PART

I

INTRODUCTION

CHAPTER 1

COMMUNITY RESPONSE

One way to stop wanderers is take away their shoes. It is certainly better than tying them to a chair. But Fred is determined. If you give him his pants, he is gone. Sonya is a repeater. Everyone on the emergency room staff knows her well. She comes to the emergency room to bathe and wash her clothes. One night a nurse found her naked at the ladies' room sink, doing her laundry. Kate has been in the mental hospital for two years. The staff considers her to be the sanest person on the ward. Unfortunately, she has too much money to be eligible for Medicaid, and she refuses to pay for nursing home placement. So she stays where she is.

Social planners have admired two decades of decentralization and deinstitutionalization as a service for the benefit of clients. The performance of human service institutions has in the past been the object of public criticism. Total institutions (mental hospitals) were criticized for dehumanizing their residents. Centralized institutions with complex procedures, structures, and bureaucracies were felt to be too inaccessible and complicated for the average patient to negotiate. A new community focus would make traditional services more accessible and responsive to the "target" population, and deinstitutionalization of state mental hospitals was accomplished in the name of community mental health. Neighborhood health centers have decentralized the primary medical care once provided solely by the city hospitals (Anderson 1974); welfare services can now be obtained at the local office. These efforts were furthered by the addition of entirely new enterprises, such as home care, meals-on-wheels, and senior citizens centers for the elderly. It was felt that bringing services to the community and thereby preserving natural supports would produce new therapeutic returns for practitioners and realize economies in financing for the politician.

Nonetheless, the long-term care of the elderly thought to be mentally

3

impaired and dependent has never been satisfactorily resolved. For years the state mental hospital was a solution accepted by society. Now the community must come to terms with the management of senile elderly, without the aid of the traditional last resort. The elderly have found very little available to them in the way of community mental health services. Less than 2.5 percent of the patients treated in community-based mental health facilities are over 65 (Statistical Notes).

Elizabeth Markson (1973) complains that geriatric overplacement in state hospitals continues to be a problem owing to the absence of services in the community. Robert Butler (1970) concludes that community placement for ex-geriatric patients is a euphemism for derelict lives in the flophouses of city slums. More old people with psychiatric diagnoses are in nursing homes than in any other institutional facility. An estimated 53 percent of nursing home residents have been identified as mentally disturbed (Redick, Kramer, and Taube 1973). Nursing homes are now criticized for being minihospitals, with the same disabling effects. The entrance of profit-motivated businesses into the field has raised the specter of financial exploitation (Mendelsohn 1974). Have the changes of the 1960s and 1970s brought the promised reform, or have they perpetuated the abuses in the guise of reformation? Present-day skepticism warrants a more thorough investigation.

How have social changes altered the fate of senile elderly and the pattern of organizational response? What is the fate of the geriatric patient admitted to the state mental hospital either prior to or in spite of the community mental health alternative? What becomes of the candidates for admission who are rejected, and must seek help elsewhere? How do social agents in the community respond now that the state mental hospital is no longer available? How can they meet their obligations to maintain, control, and treat the confused elderly? Under what circumstances are the forces of social authority activated, and how do professionals choose from among optional interventions? These important social questions have not yet been answered, after two decades of reform.

Even though social planners treat community care as an operational entity, the community is rarely the unit of analysis in research. This case study of Claiborne reconstructs a single community's response to senile dementia, and illustrates major themes in the management of dependents. In Claiborne, 15 specific locales of action within or servicing the community have been identified, as well as 223 social agents (persons in authority) and other participants (the elderly presumed senile, and those who encounter them but do not exercise authority over them). The principal service stations identified are Central State Hospital, a state mental hospital; the Geriatric Specialist Team, a community mental health center component with geriatric responsibility; City Hospital, a general medical hospital; and some nursing homes. For a complete listing, see the Appendix.

The author was directly involved in the community as a participant-observer, trying to integrate himself unobtrusively into the culture of various settings, and thereby gain firsthand knowledge of the actors' ideas and actions. Respondents were interviewed in detail about their points of view. Social factors affecting their perspectives and decisions were identified. Particular attention was given to social agents' specialized training, professional or non-professional status, organizational ideology and defined function, and role obligations as organization employees. In keeping with the holistic objectives of this study, all relevant settings were surveyed, and the points of view of all significant actors were impartially treated as definitions of social reality.

The focus is on empirical consequences of competing multiple definitions. Throughout the process of data collection and analysis, patterns of recurring empirical events were constantly watched for. The unstructured interviewing of significant social actors permitted an ongoing formulation and reformulation of assumptions and hypotheses. The process resulted in increasing sophistication and refinement in analysis of perspectives and patterns. The presentation of data reconstructs patterns that exist in the community and describes perspectives behind them.

The data are organized according to community stations rather than to theme. Again, the purpose is to maintain the identity and autonomy of community components, and thereby preserve a holistic picture of the community. The possible dimensions of community response are defined as maintenance, peacekeeping, and stabilization. Various components are categorized and presented according to their principal contribution to one of these three strategies.

The derivation of social policy implications begins with a holistic account of the institutional referral system. All community components participate in routing in varying degrees. Organizational determinants of routing decisions and social and economic influences are analyzed. Specific research strategies and program planning issues are delineated. The final chapter summarizes salient social policy themes.

OPERATIONAL DEFINITIONS

Senility

Senility is an ambigious construct. Practitioners are unable to draw a distinct line between senility and normal mentality in old age. One merges imperceptibly with the other. Therefore, senility is operationally defined in terms of the elderly's officially labeled mentality, institutional identity, and behavioral characteristics. Any aged person in Claiborne who has come to the attention of a professional with authority to apply the labels "senile," "senile dementia," or "organic brain" syndrome, and who has been so designated, is included in this study. Any aged person in a mental hospital, or previously in a mental hospital, and without alternative psychiatric diagnosis, is included. ("Alcoholic" and "burned-out schizophrenic" are alternative labels that would exclude an elderly person from this study.) Any aged person without an officially designated senile mentality or an institutional identity who manifests at least one of the following characteristics (adapted from Meacher 1972) is also included:

Verbal confusion—incoherent speech, tangential speech
Physical restlessness—aimless wandering, restless fiddling
Disorientation to person, situation, or place
Anormic behavior—nonconventional use of objects, nonconventional behavior, nonfunctional reiterative activities
Memory defect

In some cases the observer's judgment categorizes an elderly person as confused. For example, when an elderly lady sneaked out of a nursing home without money, clothing, or an obvious destination in mind (see Chapter 7), her lack of preparation and direction was interpreted as evidence of confusion. (Simultaneous application of three independent sets of criteria may or may not overlap. For instance, an elderly nursing home resident previously discharged from the state mental hospital may manifest none of the five characteristics, but nonetheless be accepted as confused in the study.)

Community

Community response is operationally delimited by identification and selection of an actual community. Claiborne is an identifiable section of a large metropolitan area. Approximately 16 percent of its 44,000 (1976) residents are elderly. Claiborne is a predominantly white residential community. It is basically a low income area with a pocket of wealthy homes. Approximately 30 level-three nursing homes (Medicaid-reimbursed custodial facilities) are concentrated in the area. Spacious homes built at the turn of the century in Claiborne have been efficiently converted into residential care facilities. These old houses can accommodate anywhere from 20 to 60 beds. The concentration of nursing homes also has drawn to Claiborne a large number of elderly ex-mental hospital patients.

The community is large enough to support a variety of health, mental health, and social and recreational services. Most are located within the geographical boundary of the community, and three of the four hospital facilities (City Hospital, Public Hospital, and Central State Hospital) are nearby. Fourteen specific locales of encounters and ten nursing homes were incorporated into this study. The number and function of stations selected was determined by extent of integration into the community pattern. Claiborne is small enough, and the number of participating stations few enough, that coverage can be comprehensive. The patterning of organizational exchanges is readily detectable.

The term "station" is used to identify any Claiborne setting that claims to give some service to confused elderly. "Station" is a useful concept because it is a neutral term. It does not assume or negate the validity of organizations' professed ideologies. Also, this term émphasizes the organizational commonality of traits that is essential in constructing a holistic picture of the community. The concept is particularly useful in analysis of the institutional referral systems in Chapter 10. Stations may be locally based or centrally located to serve the metropolitan area. They may be small, informal, and specialized or they may be large, complex, and bureaucratic. They all share a common trait of encountering and handling confused elderly.

Obviously, societal response can be observed in the function of formal organizations like hospitals, visiting nurse associations, and senior citizen centers. To the extent that one can generalize about behavior of friends, neighbors, and other concerned citizens who encounter confused elderly, they also constitute a dimension of societal response. They are separated, however, by their informal structure from the popular notion of an organization and of organizational behavior.

Actors

The significant social actors are categorized as either social agents or participants. The term "social agent" identifies persons who by virtue of their training or occupation excercise some authority over confused elderly. At one extreme is the psychiatrist, who can involuntarily commit a patient to the hospital. At the other extreme is the bus driver, who tells confused passengers when to get off the bus. At some point the line between no authority and a little authority is arbitrarily drawn. The term "participant" identifies all others who encounter confused elderly but do not exercise authority over them, for example, neighbors, senior citizens, and customers at a luncheonette.

CODIFICATION BY IDEOLOGY

Society's response to its problem with senile elderly is guided by either one or a combination of two principles: preserving social order and rehabilitating the individual. Community stations are invested with authority to implement corresponding strategies of maintenance, peacekeeping, and stabilization. Table 1 suggests the relationships among principles, strategies, and the community response in Claiborne.

TABLE 1

The Community Response: Principle, Strategy, Mechanism

Principle	Strategy	Clairborne Stations and Agents
	Maintenance	
Preserving social order through containment and control	Partial	Community scenes Locally organized interventions
	Total	Nursing home Royal, Autumn, Holst
	Peacekeeping	Geriatric specialists Police
Rehabilitation through treatment	Stabilization	Mental hospital Medical hospital

There are certain limitations to organizing community stations according to this typology. Some stations are devoted to both control and rehabilitation, for example, the mental hospital. From a medical-psychiatric perspective, the mental hospital is used for diagnosis and treatment of mental illness. Compulsory hospitalization, however, involves the mental hospital in containment and control. This is an issue of profound political and juridical importance because it involves the loss of civil and legal rights. Statutory schemes that delineate legal conditions of confinement try to integrate and balance two primary considerations: first, the interests of the community in protecting itself from dangerous and harmful acts committed by the mentally ill; and second, the interests of individuals in obtaining the best treatment available. From a juridical point of view, the state's right of police power for the purpose of self-protection and the state's authority as *parens patriae* to protect individuals unable to protect themselves are exercised through hospital commitment. In some states, the question of compulsory hospitalization is principally a problem of personal liberty versus general security (Rock 1968). While society hopes for successful treatment of persons with mental disorders, it demands the safe custody of those institutionalized. The pressure for security is embodied in custodial customs, regulations, and traditions of state mental hospitals (Hunt 1958). In this illustration, functions of treatment and control are inextricably interwoven.

Other problems in codification arise when stations generally committed to one strategy have components that can be codified under another. Nursing homes, for example, have recreational activities that are as conducive to rehabilitation as to maintaining social order. When a 94-year-old confused lady rides a roller coaster on a nursing home outing to an amusement park, the event defies classification. Also, the precision in definition of strategies is variable. The above typology of principles and strategies could be elaborated and refined. This level of precision, however, reflects the range and frequency of social interventions actually observed in Claiborne. The risk of loss of information through simplifying is compensated for by the theoretical convenience and clarity of these generalizations.

Maintenance Strategies

Provision of custodial care is the basic purpose of all maintenance strategies. Stations' resources may be allocated either to direct custodial handling of confused elderly individuals or to supporting, educating, and assisting custodial care workers. Ideally, the first objective is to maintain the elderly in their own homes (Cohen 1974), thereby preserving informal maintenance provided by family, neighbors, and friends. Visiting nurses, homemakers, outreach workers, and private physicians contribute to this effort. Failure of the home maintenance approach activates total maintenance strategies, generally nursing home placement. Basic survival needs—food, shelter, medical care, and money—are provided under supervision of the institution. Claiborne maintenance resources are enumerated in Table 2.

TABLE 2
Maintenance Work

Maintenance Stations and Agents	Official Purpose
Family	Natural support mechanism
Nursing home	Total maintenance
Senior citizen center	Food and recreation
Main Street luncheonette	Private enterprise
Geriatric outreach worker	Coordination of maintenance agents
Religious Council	Community organizer, political activism
Family counseling	Case work
Nursing home organizer	Patients' rights advocacy
Senior workshop	Sheltered employment
Welfare department	Taxi slips and homemaker approval

Peacekeeping Strategies

The peacekeepers consider senile elderly to be harmless and fragile, but sometimes disorderly and disruptive nuisances. Any disorderly conduct is attributed to confusion, not to malicious or criminal intent, therefore obviating the need for punishment. However, any confused elderly person who does not or cannot mend his disruptive ways is subject to progressively stringent enforcement of orderly conduct.

Peacekeepers undertake surveillance of areas with a concentration of confused elderly—nursing homes, senior citizen centers, the business district on Main Street. They also respond to complaints and requests for assistance. The elderly, however, are without social power to legitimize complaints, and consequently are unable to mobilize peacekeepers on their behalf. Peacekeepers disregard their claims that their disruptive behavior is a consequence of mistreatment by others, such as neighbors, family, or nursing home staff. Their stories are considered to be unreliable products of their confusion. Peacekeepers are committed to protecting their constituencies by suppressing annoyances caused by confused elderly.

In contrast to the large number of maintenance stations with specifically defined functions, there are only two peacekeeping stations, but these have diversified activities (see Table 3).

TABLE 3
Peacekeeping

Agents	Official Purpose
Geriatric specialist team	Surveillance, controlling management problems in nursing homes, securing harmonious interorganizational relations
Police	Transporting confused elderly, protecting the community

Stabilization Strategies

With the exception of some interorganizational components, treatment is the prevailing ideology in mental and medical hospitals. These stations share a common perception of organic brain deterioration as the cause of confusion in the elderly. A theoretical corollary concludes that this condition is irreversible, and that treatment for the purpose of recovery would be a futile exercise. Therefore, treatment methods are useful for retarding further deterioration or stabilizing at the present level of impairment. Treatment strategies for the confused elderly are more accurately defined as stabilization strategies (see Table 4).

It should be noted that other medical and mental health professionals at work in similar settings have been classified under maintenance and peacekeeping strategies. For example, the similarity in functioning and staffing of a neighborhood health center might warrant its classification with the medical hospital. A major objective of neighborhood health centers is maintaining patients in the community. The station, therefore, is classified as a community maintenance strategy. Also, hospitalization is the key medical strategy for stabilization; this function is unavailable at health centers.

Stabilization strategies in the medical hospital focus on controlling physical illness, disease, infection, injury, and so on. By improving the physical condition, the staff expects patients to be stabilized at an optimal level of mental functioning given the neurological impairment.

In the mental hospital, stabilizing means regulating medication. This generally implies an increase in the patient's tranquilizer dosage. A sometimes massive increase with a potential for deleterious side effects, including death, necessitates constant monitoring of changes in the patient's physical condition and behavior, as well as frequent dosage readjustments.

TABLE 4
Stabilization

Stations	Official Purpose
Mental hospital	
Admissions clinic	Screening: admission, referral
Inpatient service	Regulate medication, monitor
After-care	Prevent rehospitalization
Medical hospital	
Emergency room	Screening: admission, patient distribution, rejection
Medical ward	Recover physical health, hold until placement
Social services	Arrange for public financing
Continuing care unit	Remove patient from hospital

ROUTING DILEMMA

Once the senile elderly individual has entered the constellation of servicing stations, the timing and direction of movement from station to station are dominated by social agents. The elderly's contribution is subordinated to professional judgments. Routing decisions are, according to professionals, technical mental-medical problems of matching needs and services. There are, however, uncertainties underlying this perspective.

Convinced that the confused elderly's condition is irreversible, many stations regard their handling as a waste of scarce resources: "No one wants anyone who doesn't have potential" (nurse 3, medical ward, CH).* Stations prohibit the entrance of elderly suspected of being "managment problems." Those whose nonconventional behavior disrupts the atmosphere of tranquility or annoys other participants will be encouraged to go elsewhere to have their needs serviced. In addition, resources for care are very limited in comparison to the demand for services. Hospital staff wants to commit its resources to those who "need them most," which generally excludes the senile.

For these reasons, all servicing stations cautiously protect their boundaries. They maintain elaborate screening and discharge devices to control the size and composition of their patient-client-resident population. As a result, some senile elderly are constantly in motion, displaced from one station to another, and interorganizational associations suffer. The routing perspective of a station more often competes than conforms with that of another. Generally, there is no mutual agreement as to the meaning or motive of routing decisions made at other stations.

---

*In this and all subsequent quotes, the following abbreviations are used: CH, City Hospital; CHC, Community Health Center; CMHC, Community Mental Health Center; CSH, Central State Hospital; CSO, Community Service Organization; GST, Geriatric Specialist Team; NHC, Neighborhood Health Center; PH, Public Hospital.

2

MULTIPLE SOCIAL
DEFINITIONS

The application of labels, such as senile dementia, and the nature of subsequent social intervention are best conceived of as exchanges between actors and organizations. Understanding these exchanges begins with a search for empirical regularities in the pattern. A thorough reconstruction of social reality must go beyond this, however, to examine the motives of actors and the emotions they attach to their actions. This is accomplished by reconstructing social phenomenon from the point of view of the people involved in it.

Different actors have different perspectives for dealing with the same phenomenon, and therefore respond differently. For example, discrepancies in perspective are frequently revealed in the movement of elderly between organizations. What the staff at one station considers an "appropriate referral" may be viewed as a "dump job" at another station. In the following example, the state hospital staff member's interpretation of a confused elderly lady's behavior is determined in part by his attitude towards a second agency:

> We got a call from the state rehab agency saying that Mary sleeps while she's there, so shouldn't be given a massive dosage of tranquilizers. I'll reduce it, but I think she's just bored out there. That's why she falls asleep. (psychiatric resident 8, CSH)

The existence and use of alternative definitions by agents and participants are documented in the following.

> Senior citizen 7: Wasn't she disturbed?
> Senior citizen 8: We're all disturbed. We're normal until someone catches us in the act.

They say she's senile, but she managed to escape from the hospital and get
home. She can't be that bad. (activities director, Holst Nursing Home)

This is a confused lady, but it's an even more confused situation. (social
worker 3, CSH)

Every time I think of a characteristic of senility, I can think of an alternative
explanation. (nurse, CHC)

It should be emphasized that the task of elucidating multiple perspectives
in no way implies that one of them can or will be found to be true according
to some objective scientific standard. This study does examine, however, who
has the power to define social realities according to his particular perspective
and to make that definition prevail throughout the constellation of participating organizations.

The social agents' perspectives are determined by professional (or so-
called nonprofessional) training, by the employing station's self-defined social
function and the employees' organizational roles and by the organizational
needs of the station. Other social scientists have made similar observations.*
Melvyn Susser (1968) concluded that the culture of a medical unit influences
the practitioner's perspective for assessing a patient's needs and delivering
appropriate treatment. A nurse at a large general medical hospital who was
responsible for posthospitalization placement of confused elderly talked about
"a cute little level three." In other words, she had given a confused elderly
gentleman a social identity and name that expressed her occupational relationship to him. To this placement worker he was a "placement," not a "patient."
In response to the unconventional behavior of a confused elderly lady in the
City Hospital emergency room, a medical resident (5) revealed a biological
perspective when he described her as "a little frontal lobish." The interaction
of these variables as they form perspectives and contribute to the decisions and
actions of social agents is elaborated in Chapters 3 through 12.

PATHOLOGY AND PROFESSIONALS

It is useful to introduce at this point, in general terms, two basic frames
of reference for defining and interpreting senile behavior and cognition. This
previews the methodological approach of this study, and demonstrates the

---

*These concepts have also been applied to the study of delinquents (Fabricant 1975) and
alcoholics (Wiseman 1970).

possibility of multiple and contradicting interpretations of the same "facts." The first point of view, one taken by most professionals, characterizes senility as a pathological condition from which no one recovers. A second and contrasting point of view, formulated by other participants and a minority of professionals, hold that, though certain behavior and cognition remain incomprehensible and violate customary social norms, "senile" characteristics may be products of personal resourcefulness rather than pathology.

Dependency and fragility are general attributes ascribed to senile elderly.

They can no longer repress dependency needs. They are like children who demand immediate help and gratification. (social worker 2, CSH)

Old people are fragile, both in a medical and emotional sense. If they get sick, they may become depressed; if they are depressed, it can make them sick. These people are also vulnerable in a social sense; they are easy prey for muggers. And on the service (Central State Hospital) old people are just slow moving targets in a fast moving place. (psychiatric resident 5, CSH)

Behind a manifest resistance is likely to lie a latent wish to be cared for, protected, and helped. (Wasser 1971)

The majority of professionals also share a belief that senility is a chronically stable impairment, that, whatever the cause, the condition is irreversible:

Nobody can cure old age, not social intervention or whatever intervention. (psychiatric social worker, CH)

No one has ever seen a senile dementia reversed. (medical resident, CH)

True senility is unremittable, irreversible. (psychiatrist, GST)

Given the futility of treatment implicit in these professionals' perspective, senility is a very serious pathology. Yet the term is casually equated with aging, and is used as a catchall to identify dependent, deviant behavior. It is generally but not universally recognized that not all elderly are senile. For example, some professionals choose to make a distinction between "true" aging and "chronological" aging (Goldfarb 1974). In other words, mental and physical decline is the definition of being old. The nondisabled are considered either exceptions or not truly aged. V. A. Kral (1970) defines the age period of 65 and over as "senescence," and differentiates between benign and malignant senescence.

We all get senile sooner or later; it's just a matter of time. (psychiatric resident 1, CSH)

> I don't have any direct contact with elderly. I do see one 94-year-old lady but I don't consider her elderly. Her mental facilities are intact. (community worker, NHC)

> Everybody is senile to a certain degree. I'm a little forgetful. (head nurse, Holst Nursing Home)

When "true" aging is seen as synonymous with pathological deterioration, any chronologically aged person is a likely candidate for the senility label. Even though professionals claim to diagnose senility on the basis of a standardized measure, the mental status exam, in practice their diagnosis is the "professionalization" of senility in its common usage. The label is applied to any forgetful, disoriented, down-and-out old person:

> Anyone who is disoriented and not expected to improve is called demented. (nurse 1, medical ward, CH)

> People who are old and worn out are called senile. (nurse 2, emergency room, CH)

> She is old, lonely and confused. I guess she's senile. (social worker 5, CH)

According to medical and mental health doctrines, "senility," "dementia," "senile dementia," and "organic brain syndrome" are diagnostic categories applied in accordance with certain indicators called symptoms. Determination of symptomatic behavior is usually limited to measurement of the individual's biological, cognitive, or emotional state. The defect lies somewhere in the makeup of the individual (Spitzer and Denzin 1968). Professionals in the field also use these diagnostic categories to identify old people who do not take proper care of themselves, at least according to conventional standards. The elderly's daily maintenance habits, sociability, and conventionality are integral parts of the applied configuration of senility. One dimension of the expanded symptom concept is labeled the "tea and toast" syndrome.

> An elderly lady lives alone in an apartment. She loses her taste for food, and eats only toast. She develops vitamin deficiencies. She doesn't drink enough fluids, and becomes dehydrated. She soon becomes confused, and is brought to the hospital. (psychiatric resident 1, CSH)

> The most typical case is of the elderly widowed lady who just survives on her social security, and lives alone. There is no real responsive next of kin. It's the tea and toast syndrome. (psychiatrist, PH)

A similar notion, which reflects the apparent social isolation, is called the "little old lady (LOL)" syndrome.

We call it the Little Old Lady syndrome. They are old, dying, and no one cares. We had one old lady who called at three every morning. We'd go up and visit. She was just lonesome, and wanted someone to talk to. (ambulance driver, CH)

They don't have social contacts. They only watch television, and cook meals on a hot plate. (social worker, CH)

She was living alone. She had no living relatives. Her last living son died, and her television broke down. She lost even the "soapies." (psychiatric nurse 1, CSH)

The professionals' view of the plight of nursing home residents does not substantially differ from their generalizations about the functional inadequacy and isolation of the senile living at home. Restrictive institutional environments of nursing homes discourage social interaction and suppress self-expression (Lieberman 1974). Residents feel sad, lonely, and abandoned. They are without stimulation or involvement in contemporary events. Even though their daily needs may be managed for them, the environmental symptoms prevail. Residence in a nursing home has even become an indicator of senility.

The majority of professionals draw a pathetic picture of the senile elderly, who are described as weak, defeated, and fragile. They may neglect even the most elementary survival needs. They are chronic "noncopers" and the victims of "some miserable blows in life." They suffer "some sort of degenerative syndrome" from which there is no recovery. Whether they live in a private residence or in a nursing home, their life circumstances are essentially the same —miserable. Senility is psychologically equaled with despair.

ETIOLOGIC UNCERTAINTY

When social agents plan intervention strategies, one question invariably arises: What causes senility? If causes can be discovered and eradicated by appropriate intervention, then the problem will vanish. The recurring inadequacy of all strategies, however, has left society and its professional agents confused about the causes and the appropriate societal response.

The professionals' ideas about the etiology of senility can be organized into four categories: organic mental disease, social isolation, combination, and celestial.

The causal explanation, the most widely accepted, assumes that senility is the result of organic impairment in the brain. Such terms as "organic deficit," "brain cell loss or dysfunction," and "wasting of neurons" are commonly used to identify the effect. Specialists also say that diminished blood flow to the brain is associated with the organic change. This might be a result of hardening of the arteries, arteriosclerosis, occluding blood vessels to the brain, arterovascular disease, or Alzheimer's disease. A second explanation assumes that senility is the result of inadequate environmental stimulation. The elderly whose lives are confined to nursing homes have no need to know the time of day, the day, or year, so they lose contact with time in general and become lost in their timeless world. Others in the community live alone, without friends or relatives. They are afraid to walk on the street, and do so only when absolutely necessary. The absence of regular human contact results in a loss of social reference. More abstractly, the condition is attributed to "sensory deprivation or too little stroking" (psych nurse 2, emergency room, CH).

The most important thing is stimulation and emotional contact. (social worker, CH)

The confused old person needs direct stimulation. Direct talk about family or recent familiar events can accomplish visible reorientation. (continuing care worker 1, CH)

There are those who integrate organic and social factors into a combination theory of etiology. Senility is the "culmination of interacting forces"— social isolation, arteriosclerosis, genetic inheritance, physiological constitution, age, and the accumulation of lifelong problems.

The inactivity and decrease in environmental stimulation, resulting from a withdrawal from surroundings, give rise to a mental deterioration process concurrently with physiological cerebral deterioration that occurs in old age. (Barnes 1974)

A final etiological theory relates senility to celestial forces.* Specifically, deviant behavior in the elderly, particularly those in nursing homes, is supposedly aroused by the appearance of a full moon. While this theory may strike the reader as blatantly antiscientific, numerous practitioners voiced confidence in its explanatory credibility. Perhaps the mere appearance of such an interpretation illustrates the etiologic uncertainty.

---

*At first glance, the reader might suspect that social agents offer such a theory tongue in cheek. However, agents from all different disciplinary backgrounds and at different levels in the professional hierarchy professed sincere belief in celestial causes. Although the notion does not appear in the literature, it nonetheless has widespread credibility in the field. In a scientific era, such celestial theories are immediately greeted with skepticism, but one must bear in mind that in comparison to other theories, it is no less reliable a predictor of deviant behavior.

On the nights of the full moon, you can always expect something. One time three people walked in here stark naked. The staff around here certainly believes in the full moon theory. (psychiatrist 2, emergency room, CH)

The full moon does it to them. But it will pass in a few days. (night supervisor, Court Nursing Home)

There *is* a full moon syndrome. (medical resident 3, CH)

Other similar notions attribute the appearance of senile characteristics to "seasonal fluctuations." Senile old people are often described as being "out of this world" or "off in their own little ether," and treatment is a matter of "bringing them down to earth."

DEFYING PROFESSIONAL CONVENTIONS

As already pointed out, the notion of senility is frequently equated with growing old. Some motor and sensory deterioration common to aging may result in peculiarities in everyday behavior that others view as evidence of confusion. An illustration frequently cited is an aged person who does not hear well, misunderstands the social agent's question, gives an erroneous answer, and is considered to be confused because of the "inappropriate" response. Removing the elderly from productive roles in the economy imposes an economic dependency that by itself is a violation of social norms (Folsom and Folsom 1974). The elderly as patients, clients, or residents are relegated to an inferior social position when dealing with doctors, nurses, and social workers (Stotsky 1970).

To the extent that professionals mimic and integrate societal discrimination, their perspective is a mechanism of social control rather than the application of scientific principles to the treatment of human beings. It prevails since old people are powerless to challenge the stereotype and to defend themselves against social agents. Under these conditions, senility is a rationalization for handling (removing) subjects of societal discrimination.

Recently I became ill in a strange city, and went to a hospital. A doctor took one look at me, and without a question or a test, pronounced me hopelessly senile. That seems to be the general attitude toward all old people. We are constantly being repressed, insulted, and humiliated simply because we are no longer young. (in Gaitz and Scott 1975)

Certain senile behavior or the behavior of those considered to be senile contradicts professional conventions, and illustrates how old people struggle to survive from a position of economic disadvantage and social inferiority. In viewing the behavior of other populations in similar circumstances (alcoholics, juvenile delinquents, New York City indigents), researchers (Wiseman 1970; Fabricant 1975; Love 1956) have successfully constructed similar alternative frameworks (see Table 5).

TABLE 5
Competing Frameworks

Pathological Stereotypes	Resourceful Strategies
Chronically stable, irreversible	Fluctuation, improvement
Weak, defeated	Tenacious, defiant
Disorganized, incompetent	Clever, calculating, manipulative

Although there is widespread agreement that the senile condition is stable and irreversible, the hospital staff acknowledges that continual fluctuation in behavior of senile patients complicates the referral process. Nursing home administrators often complain that hospital staff has described inaccurately a patient's condition. Placement workers must reassess a patient's condition as close as possible to time of discharge.

> Very sudden and dramatic changes do occur in the older person's mental status. (continuing care worker 2, CH)

> She looked like a classic senile confused case but she came out of it. (continuing care worker, 2, PH)

> There was one old man here who was really obnoxious. He was here two years. He had been some sort of traffic engineer, and on the ward he spent his days giving directions to pedestrian traffic. He was always urinating in the waste baskets, and defecating on the floor. One day he was unusually quiet, and that night he said, "I'm going to bed." That was the first time in two years he had gone to bed without a struggle. The next day he asked, "Where's the bathroom?" We were shocked. He was discharged a week later. No one knew what happened or why he changed so suddenly. (psychiatric nurse 12, CSH)

Misdiagnosis is a common professional explanation to account for supposedly impossible improvement in the senile condition. Any old person whose confusion improves or disappears was not truly senile. The prevailing conception of senility goes unchallenged. "The psychiatrist admitted an elderly lady. He diagnosed her senile. She's on the medical ward now, doing just fine" (psych nurse 3, emergency room, CH).

Senile elderly are invariably described as mentally and physically weak, "biding their time between heaven and hell". Even under the most oppressive circumstances, however, elderly identified as senile have demonstrated an indomitable spirit:

[An elderly gentleman on the orthopedic ward at City Hospital was barely able to talk.]
Nurse: Did you like the nursing home?
Man [with clenched fist]: No, because they took away my freedom.

The nursing home staff made him throw something out. He climbed in the dumpster to get it. They refused to let him keep it. He refused to come out. They were really upset, like he was doing something immoral, being in a dumpster. Finally they gave in, and let him keep it. It was the only way they could get him out. (neighbor, Claiborne)

She is stubborn, independent, and uncooperative. She does what she wants, and when she says, "No," it's like a brick wall. (staff nurse, Brady Nursing Home)

A sense of personal disorder and inability to manage daily needs in a purposeful way is frequently attributed to the elderly. Many of the elderly labeled senile, however, demonstrate imaginative and resourceful survival strategies, as well as mental acuity for environmental contingencies:

She kept her fur coat in a trash can so that it wouldn't be stolen. (family counselor 1, CSO)

She tells customers in restaurants that she is starved, and they buy her meals. Once the waitress refused her order, telling the customer, "I've already served her one breakfast this morning." (staff nurse, Brady Nursing Home)

If you buy her shoes, she sells them, and spends the money on what she wants. (staff nurse, Brady Nursing Home)

Attempts to make supposedly senile patients take medication against their will are likely to elicit professional recognition of their cleverness: "She won't take her medication. She's too smart. She won't even let me follow her into the bathroom after the medication rounds" (staff nurse, Bank Nursing Home). Sometimes distinguishing between confusion and cleverness is impossible: "She can't keep her mind on what you want her to do. You don't know if she is being crafty or really can't remember" (staff nurse, Bank Nursing Home).

When social agents suspect that disordered and confused behavior is purposeful rather than purposeless, they identify the elderly person as a con artist, as well as senile, without the slightest reservation. It is apparently less complicated to embrace incongruence than to challenge professional assumptions: "She's sly like a fox, and that's the hardest kind to work with. She's a con artist. She plays up her weakness" (psychiatric nurse 2, GST).

An obvious cleverness is demonstrated in attempts to manipulate social agents and organizations without appearing to do so:

> [An elderly lady diagnosed as senile wanted to be admitted to City Hospital. She told the admitting officer]: I have aneurism and a heart condition. You ought to let me in. (Louise)

> He got some money from the nursing home for new shoes, and spent it on something else. Then he complained at the senior citizen center about his shoes. The director bought him a new pair, and sent the bill to the home. He is cagey. (psychiatric nurse 1, GST)

Finally, there are some who realize the advantage of making a good bargain, and are willing to lay their cards on the table.

> A crazy, senile 76-year-old lady used to come in here all the time. The first thing she said to me was, "I write letters." What she meant was that she writes to the administration declaring her appreciation for the good service delivered by. . . . I couldn't help but respond to this. Such letters are very important in this hospital. They get so many complaints that any commendation is taken seriously. Doctors who get such letters receive the best residencies, so it's very important to them. (social worker 5, CH)

To the vast majority of professionals, senile behavior is pathological. Qualities attributed to this pathology are irreversible disability, defeated spirit, and purposeless behavior. The same behavior can also be viewed as evidence of personal resourcefulness. Some senile elderly are even recognized as con artists. Because an old person wanders away from a nursing home and gets lost doesn't mean that he or she didn't have a good time or that the outing accomplished no purpose. The senile are capable of holding tenaciously to their ideals. Which frame of reference, pathology or resourcefulness, is true? In the absence of convincing etiologic evidence, neither has a claim to superior truth. Supported by societal conventions and social authority invested in professional human caretakers, the pathological perspective dominates.

The terms "senile dementia," "dementia," and "organic brain" syndrome are used interchangeably to define individualistic conditions (biological and psychic diseases) and environmental situations. In fact, the terms are used to identify all varieties of dependent and nonconventional behavior. Senility takes into account the residual deviant behavior left unexplained by all other causative factors. (Thomas Scheff [1966] proposed a similar construct of residual deviance.) Because the word "senility" has so many uses in the field, and because its use presupposes the authenticity of a particular perspective, it is the author's preference to subsume all those conditions popularly and professionally spoken of as senility under the generic term "confusion." In the remainder of the book, the term "confused elderly" is substituted for senile and other professionally used terms.

3

IN THE COMMUNITY

There is a small social space for confused elderly that is uninhabited by professional social agents. Confused elderly commonly appear on the main streets of Claiborne, in public places and commercial establishments, and at public events. They encounter citizens on the street and families at home.

STREET SCENES

Street scenes are not limited to the literal street. As a category of deviant behavior, they can be performed in a public library, on the bus, in the post office, in the park, or any other public place. All the following street scenes are regularly recurring events, and some are dramatic enough to elicit an immediate response from spectators. When the audience or spectators play an active part, their responses will also be noted.

The most notorious of the street performers is Sonya, the "bag lady." (The bag lady is a characterization developed by Sharon Curtin.) She carries all her possessions with her in two plastic bags, and claims City Park as her residence. Her costuming is spectacular. Visible are the hemlines of at least three dresses; the outermost is a brilliant red velvet. She wears several sweaters and a heavy coat over the dresses. To the City Hospital staff, she is both a colorful eccentric and a nuisance:

She's not on welfare because she has no address. She won't stay anywhere long enough to receive a welfare check. (social worker 1, CH)

Once we undressed her, and found cheese and a roll of salami. (nurse 2, emergency room, CH)

The story is that she was giving some workmen in a street manhole a hard time. They weren't too pleasant themselves, so she just lifted up her skirts, and dumped on them right there. (nurse 1, emergency room, CH)

Less glamorous performers on the street become socially visible when they are recognized for a single idiosyncratic characteristic. The following are illustrative street names used by spectators to identify specific old people:

... Coughin' Annie (chef, Main Street Luncheonette). ... the Cryer—She spends all day feeding pigeons and crying (chef, luncheonette). ... the Picker —The old guy comes in here every day. He spends about an hour going through the barrels. If he finds anything of obvious value, he returns it to us. I guess he's just looking for something to do, and it's safer and warmer in here than out on the street (clerk, post office). ... Faith, Hope and Charity —You never see those three crazy characters apart (chef, Main Street luncheonette). ... the Prop—He'd come in wearing his VFW garrison hat, and hang around all day leaning on the counter (clerk, post office). ... the Machine—She carries around that sewing machine everywhere she goes. She says if she left it at home, someone would steal it (senior citizen center director 1). ... Speedy—We call him Speedy because he moves so slow (chef, luncheonette). ... the Night Watchman—He walks the streets all night. About two A.M. he's at the fire station getting coffee, then at four he's over at the post office, and by six the luncheonette is open so he goes there (policeman 1).

The city-government-sponsored events for seniors also provide staging and large audiences for the street scenes:

At a sing-a-long in the park, Elvira showed up wearing an extravagant hat. Her slip hung under her dress, both brassiere straps hung down on her shoulders, her hair was dishevelled, and she smelled. She complained that she'd been evicted from her house, and that kids had stolen her money. She bummed food, and stashed it in her bag. The other seniors paid her deliberate inattention. (observation)

At a seniors' picnic that drew thousands of elderly, and provided no toilets, an elderly lady was seen positioning herself between two metal folding chairs. She raised her dress, and relieved herself. (observation)

Panhandling is the most frequent of the street scenes. It is a performance that draws the spectator into the scene. Some elderly panhandlers are considered dangerous; others, a minor nuisance.

There's nothing else for them to do but bum cigarettes. It's a kind of social exchange. (customer 1, luncheonette)

I gave him a quarter, and said, "Now don't tell, or they'll all be after me." (customer 2, luncheonette)

There's one mean one. If you don't give him cigarettes, he'll ask for money. He steals candy from little children. Or he waits for them to come out of the candy store, and takes their change (customer 3, luncheonette)

The panhandler sees himself as engaged in a legitimate economic pursuit, and victimized by the local authorities' occasional harassment.

I only get one dollar a week from the nursing home. They wouldn't even give me money for a haircut. I make about two dollars a day. It used to be better but a police detective caught me, and said if he saw me doing it again, he'd throw me in the clinker. So now I just go up and down the side streets. (panhandler)

Some street scenes are best categorized according to the spectator's setting. The firemen, in this respect, successfully portray the part of audience. On warm days they take their place beside the fire house, a few feet from the sidewalk. They play their part enthusiastically, commenting on the passersby. Though most of their attention is focused on youth and women, they also related interactions with confused elderly:

Most of them are just lonely. They'll talk to you all day if you let them. I try to avoid them. (fireman 1)

They like to talk to people in uniform. It gives them a sense of recognition. It makes them feel good. (fireman 1)

The public transit system provides Claiborne with a special minibus that makes a loop through the community every 20 minutes. Both drivers and riders are regulars. Confused elderly also make their appearance on this revolving stage:

A mumbling elderly lady climbed on the bus, and asked me to move. "I'm gonna have both my feet amputated. The doctor says it's gangrene." Before I could move, she walked to the back of the bus. (observation)

Bus driver [to a confused elderly lady]: Come on, get off here. This is your stop. My God, someday you're gonna kill yourself.

The quiet of a public library and the potentially large audience provide another opportunity for the confused elderly performer:

An elderly lady was surrounded by 40 or 50 people, and she addressed them in a hysterical voice, "Oh, my God, you're not safe anywhere. You wouldn't believe what they did to me. Even a doctor wouldn't believe it." To the police who arrived a short time later, she reported that her purse had been stolen. When the police questioned her further, she was vague and unresponsive; she even refused to give her name and address. They finally convinced her to accompany them to the police station where they would "file a complaint." The lady's performance as a victim was flawed. No one witnessed the criminal act. No one knew what happened. The police didn't investigate. No witnesses were sought. Her hysteria appeared exaggerated. A librarian concluded, "The lady has gone off the deep end." (observation)

The luncheonette on Main Street is a private business enterprise with a largely working class and retired working class clientele. Many of the regulars are nursing home residents and employees. When nursing home employees come down the street looking for stray residents, they always check first at the luncheonette.

The luncheonette is owned and managed by the chef and his family. When questioned about their reasons for servicing a confused elderly clientele that does not spend much money and may drive away better paying customers, their answers were vague and elusive. The notion of social responsibility contributes less to their perspective than does a political-economic ideology upholding consumer sovereignty and democracy. Whether it is the chef's influence or their own personal perspectives, the other patrons share the management's tolerance. Association with those in a state of diminished social grace is more a way of life than an isolated event to be managed:

> There but for the grace of God go I. That's what I always say. (customer 3)

> I hope and pray my mind don't go on me. It's a terrible thing when that happens, when it breaks. There's nothing you can do about it. (customer 4)

The patrons know and use the colloquial titles given the confused elderly: the Cryer, the Night Watchman, and so on. They exchange stories with one another about the latest episodes involving these elderly. Unconventional behavior is viewed as curious and eccentric rather than graceless and profaning. The stories told by patrons and the owners emphasize the humorous rather than pathetic aspects of the confused elderly's lives:

> He takes half an hour to order. Then he says, "Hurry up with that order. I got a lot to do." (chef)

THE FAMILY

There is a classic conception of the family as one of the "natural" channels through which an individual's needs are properly met. Likewise, it is implied that the failure of this institution under certain circumstances necessitates societal intervention, for example, the mental hospital or the nursing home. A decline of the family as a natural resource for old people is attributed to industrialization (Wilensky and Lebeaux 1965). The shift from agricultural self-sufficiency to the factory system displaced the elderly as meaningful economic and social contributors to the family. With industrialization came the emancipation and migration of adult children. Aged parents are left alone (Parsons 1949).

This notion of the "stranded" (Wilensky and Lebeaux 1965) aged parent is now in dispute. Today, social scientists are more likely to point out that the elderly family still exists and that intergenerational dislocation is not as extensive as once thought. Evidence that the family still survive can be taken from Bureau of Census data. Seventy percent of the elderly are members of at least a two-person family (see Table 6). As for dislocation, in one study of nine midwestern states, 80 percent of those elderly interviewed had living children in the same neighborhood, and one-third had brothers or sisters within 25 miles (Hansen et al. 1965). In Marjorie Lowenthal's community survey (1967), 46 percent of the elderly lived within an hour's drive of at least one child.

TABLE 6
Living Patterns of the Elderly, 1970

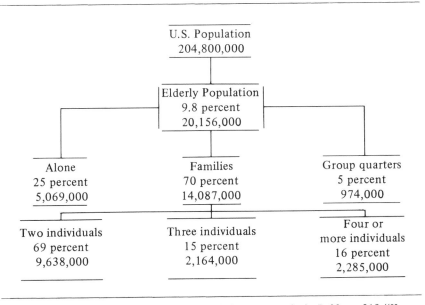

Source: U.S. Bureau of Census, Current Population Reports: Series P-20, no. 218, "Household and Family Characteristics," March 1970, Table 10; and Series P-20, no. 212, "Marital Status and Family Status," March 1970, Tables 2, 6.

This "rediscovery" of the American elderly family, plus the deinstitution-alization of the state mental hospital and the return of many confused elderly to the community, has stimulated professional interest in the family as an overlooked maintenance resource. Do confused elderly have access to kinship? Are families willing or able to maintain them, and for how long and under what circumstances?

It is a frequent observation of professionals from all settings that the confused elderly they encounter are without family, or at least without partic-ipating family. In fact, the appearance of a confused older person is often attributed to the absence of family:*

> There are either few elderly with families or a lot of elderly with no visiting family. (social worker 1, CH)

> The old people who end up at Central State Hospital or in nursing homes are people without families. That is part of why they appear. (welfare wor-ker 3)

> We rarely have home care services for discharged state mental hospital geriatric patients. Most of them have exhausted any family resources by the time they reach the hospital. (welfare worker 3)

When families do bring elderly members to professional managers, it is be-cause, from their point of view, they are overburdened and near exhaustion. They have done what they could, but they need help. This characterization is supported by families, occasionally by professionals in the field, and in the literature.

> She calls up the police, and says I mistreat the children, and that my husband runs around with other women. I can't keep her at home any more; she is destructive. (family member)

> Her mother has the choice between the two daughters. With one daughter, she helps out around the house, does dishes, even contributes to the rent. But she won't stay there. She insists on staying with Sandy who is really op-pressed. She has an eight-week-old daughter. She doesn't have enough money to pay her expenses, and her mother refuses to help. We arranged a

---

*A word of caution is in order. The stable family that successfully maintains a confused elderly member is undetected in this study. This is an obvious bias toward the problem family, and therefore the data are generalizable. Furthermore, the more insulated professionals are from the community, the less they know about or explore the family situation. Their accounts of family attendance are at times uninformed and speculative.

placement, but Sandy changed her mind at the last minute. She felt guilty. Her sister only encourages her guilt by saying their mother would die in a nursing home. (family counselor 1)

The surfacing of the confused elderly is primarily associated with the absence of family or with the exhausted family. The family appears seeking professional maintenance help through placement, generally in a nursing home. Placement is a last resort, preceded by alternative solutions that brought severe economic, personal, and social stress to the family (Lowenthal 1967; Whitehead 1970).

There are some families whose participation is deemed undesirable. Continued participation may be more deleterious to the confused elderly's well-being than the family's absence.

My husband is an ex-state hospital patient himself. We were living together for a while. When I started breaking things up around the house, he called me into the bedroom, and chained me to the bed. He brought me a can for you know . . . but I wouldn't use it. My daughter snuck me food. The time before I was really confused and didn't know what he was doing, but this time I wasn't so bad. I started sweet talkin' him so that he would let me go. [Her association with Central State Hospital began when her daughter was admitted for attempted suicide.] (Bertha)

I took my mother to visit him [the respondent's father who was admitted to a general hospital for the purpose of placement]. They held hands. He recognized her but couldn't speak to her. Now I don't know if I should have taken her. She seems worse, more upset than ever, after visiting him. (daughter)

The Professional Response

The professionals in the field rarely have extensive contact with the families of confused elderly. They frequently accuse the families of neglecting their elderly members. In fact, the appearance of the confused elderly is considered evidence of that neglect.

Families bring in old people who are bizarre, and want them committed. (psych nurse 3, emergency room, CH)

The hardest people to get involved with the patient is the family. (head nurse, Court Nursing Home)

Louie has a large family, all doctors and lawyers. I called someone in his family every day for two weeks. They always promised but never came.

Finally one son came twice, and that was it. (head nurse, Court Nursing Home)

Some confused elderly make the same accusations of their family:

I have four children, and I haven't seen one of them in 40 years. (Ed, resident, Court Nursing Home)

My daughter has forgotten me. She and her husband got my money. I don't have a cent. (Frank, patient, CSH)

Neglect is not the only criticism of the families. Some are accused of taking advantage of, even abusing, their confused elderly member:

She has good reason to be bitter. Her family stole her estate. They had her declared legally incompetent, committed her to the hospital, and took all her money. (social worker 3, CSH)

The usual family visit is once a month when the patient's personal allowance check comes in. (head nurse, Court Nursing Home)

Her niece was keeping her Veteran's and Social Security check. She refused to turn them over to the nursing home. She refused to take her aunt back even though she wants to leave. (nursing home administrator, Thompson chain)

When families think of themselves as burdened, and professionals in the field think of them as neglectful or abusive, it is no wonder that their relationship is adversarial while supposedly cooperative. The active family may disapprove of the way an elderly member is being handled, and the managers find the family uncooperative about placement problems.

Disinterested families are not likely to question the handling of the confused elderly person, but they often present problems to placement staff. Either the family refuses to take responsibility for placement or it opposes the staff's placement decisions:

We told the family we wanted to place him in a nursing home. They said, "He's too sick. We're going to call our congressman. If anything happens, you're responsible." They refused to take care of him. We had no choice. (intern, emergency room, CH)

The order of responsibility is reversed from what it should be. Now the responsibility for placement belongs to the treaters. The family is in a position to veto, not to help. I tell them, "Remember, we are helping you; you aren't helping us." Sometimes a miniconfrontation is necessary. (psychiatrist, PH)

CHAPTER

4

LOCALLY ORGANIZED
INTERVENTION

Many social agents may be involved in handling a single confused elderly person. An individual enters the community chain if he or she becomes visible to surveillance workers or if he or she is referred to a community agency like the Visiting Nurse Association (VNA) on discharge from City or Public Hospital. A confused elderly person is removed from the chain by relocation to a new area, by institutionalization, or by death.

While some of the community work is conducted as a simple one-shot encounter, such as filling out a public housing application or a nursing home consultation, most of it is more complex. A confused elderly person usually has maintenance problems that cannot be quickly resolved. The problems are not easily categorized in terms of the professional disciplines or the defined functions of the stations.

The following cases are best defined generically as community problems because of the range of maintenance difficulties presented. They illustrate the fundamentals of doing community maintenance work.

He's diabetic and alcoholic. He exposes himself, uses abusive language, and is combative. He wears a prosthesis. Central State Hospital threw him out of the inpatient service for drinking on the ward. We've placed him in public housing next to a VNA station. And were they mad about that. I manage his money even though I'm not the legal conservator. We involved an OEO agency, the surplus food program, home care, the VNA heavily, Public Hospital, and Senior Services. It's been time consuming but he's shown great progress. It doesn't always work out so well. (family counselor 1)

He's been in and out of mania all his life. He held a civil service position and couldn't be fired, so he was continually demoted. He's become increasingly demented. The social worker has known him for 20 years. Once he was admitted to the hospital against his will, and held for two weeks until a workup could be completed. His children won't have anything to do with him. I'm sure he's been very difficult to live with all these years. His wife calls every day. She can't handle him anymore. During the day he has few problems, but at night he wanders. The police have picked him up. He's a threat to himself. Nursing homes refuse to take this kind of wanderer. A state mental hospital is the only place for him, but they won't take him either. He isn't crazy enough. If I tried an involuntary commitment, and he took it to court, I could look mighty foolish. During the day he appears to be perfectly sane. Another problem is his prescription for Mellaril. He either forgets to take it or takes too many pills, so he's a potential suicide threat. There's nothing to be done for this guy. We must wait until he either dies or deteriorates further or overdoses. Then someone will get involved. (psychiatrist, CH)

There is a great diversity in Claiborne's locally organized service activities. With the exception of private physicians, these are all stations or agents whose presence is legitimated by the community care ideology. Their local activities are autonomously organized and carried out, though they all have formal or informal alliances with large institutions responsible for the entire metropolitan area. Claiborne is well supplied with such local stations and agents. The following encounter confused elderly, or at least claim to: senior citizen center, geriatric outreach, family counseling, nursing home organizer, senior workshop, welfare, neighborhood health center, and private physicians.

A SENIOR CITIZEN CENTER

The senior citizen center offers the Claiborne elderly hot meals and social and recreational activities. Backed by public funds and a human servicing ideology, centers give an outward impression of providing benevolent and sympathetic help for the community's most economically and socially disadvantaged seniors. In fact, the center is a closed society dominated by middle-class women. For them, the group luncheon is a serious social occasion. Proper conduct is narrowly defined and deviance is not tolerated. Those unable to toe the mark are forced to withdraw. The leadership is ambivalent when social responsibility and self-determination are in conflict.

Comments from marginal participants and the directors give evidence of middle-class exclusiveness:

This is a friendly place, but it all stops right here at the table. If you're not on the inside and part of the clique, well, you're left out. (senior citizen 1)

The seniors even complain about a woman who sits with her legs too far apart. But these are middle-class people, and you'll always get that sort of thing. (senior citizen center director 2)

The social worker from Central State Hospital brought in a lady who smelled. These are very clean middle-class people here, and they complained about her. (senior citizen center director 2)

Center members are most inhospitable to those confused elderly thought to be in a state of diminished social grace. Determinations of social grace are based primarily on conformity to the role of luncheon companion. Those who smell, drool, mumble, or pick at others' food are not good luncheon companions.

It's a real problem getting seniors to accept someone who drools in his lunch. (senior citizen center director 3)

He dropped his head in his food, and just stayed there like that. We can't have that. (senior citizen center director 1)

One lady mumbled all during the speaker's talk. We were so upset. (senior citizen 2)

How can I eat my lunch and sit next to someone who smells like that? (senior citizen 3)

In addition to exhibiting good table manners, male members must not display any hint of lechery:

When Jerry told me a joke about a hard-on, the others discreetly walked away. (observation)

I was so upset by the way he talked to the ladies, I finally told him, "I'm sick of you. Now keep away from me." (senior citizen 2)

The negative sanctions against lechery are particularly ironical given the degree of explicit sexual humor and conversation that is part of the insiders' gossip:

Director 1: We're collecting money to buy a new church organ.
    Senior Citizen 3: Well, don't send anyone to my door if he hasn't got an organ.

They love to gossip. They say Harriet is trying to lay Ralph. (senior citizen center director 3)

Oh, so that's why my husband's was all bent over like this. [She held up a crooked finger to demonstrate the shape of her husband's penis.] (senior citizen 6)

Diminished social grace is also measured by institutional affiliation, the most demeaning being a nursing home resident. Not one nursing home resident comes to lunch at the center even though there are two homes on the same block. Nursing home residents are stereotyped as the mumblers and droolers.

It's a real problem getting the senior citizens to accept nursing home patients. (senior citizen center director 3)

There are a lot here from the nursing homes. They're all mental, you know. (senior citizen 2)

Some of them come with social workers. That's how we know they're a little sick. (senior citizen 6)

The marginal seniors who are neither insiders nor outcasts know their survival in the center is contingent upon self-restraint:

I'm not one of those screw-loose kinds. Some people may not understand me so I don't spring my ideas on everyone. (senior citizen 7)

I occasionally talk to people about my ideas; some take it, some think I'm an agitator. (senior citizen 8)

Once those elderly with diminished social grace have been identified, they are subject to exclusionary practices:

I say hello, good-by, tell her she looks nice, but I don't have time to socialize with everyone. (senior citizen 2)

[While I was sitting on a park bench at the seniors' picnic, an elderly lady passed by looking for a place to sit and eat. I was about to offer her my seat, but the senior at my side restrained me.] Oh, don't do that! Her problem is she's not 100 percent, if you know what I mean. She picks at your plate. She'll ask for anything, and, of course, you wanting to be polite, can't tell her no. It's just awful. I don't want to be mean, but I just couldn't have her sitting here. (senior citizen 9)

As for the social obligation of senior citizen center members to accept and support confused elderly, center leaders see both pros and cons:

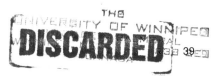

I sympathize with the seniors. This is the main meal of the day for them. They can't sit next to someone who picks food off all the plates. (senior citizen center director 1)

This is the seniors' organization. I can't make their decisions for them. (senior citizen center director 1)

They won't complain to me too much any more. I won't put up with it. If they haven't got anything better to think about, I give them something to do. (senior citizen center director 2)

You must look at it from her side too; everybody has to have friends no matter how bad they smell. (senior citizen center director 1)

Fear of being profaned by graceless associations in inescapable social settings dominates the member-outsider relationship. Once the seats at the luncheon table have been filled, the members cannot leave until the meal is finished. If their table companion is one without grace, they have no choice but to endure. Controlling the entrance and seating of confused elderly is essential to avoiding hardships. Their obligation to make sacrifices in the name of social conscience is a powerful appeal, but the right to a pleasant lunch with the companions of their choice takes precedence.

GERIATRIC OUTREACH

In Claiborne, there is a complex association of stations in which the geriatric social worker is the presiding specialist. Her position is funded by the Claiborne Outreach Clinic (which is under the financial auspices of Central State Hospital). A geriatric community organizer is cofunded by the same clinic and the Claiborne Religious Council. Both organizations contribute to the operation of a senior citizen center. The council also pays rent ($50 a week) to one of its member churches for the seniors' dining room and use of the kitchen, and rents another building for the use of the outreach team. The senior citizens' budget pays the geriatric outreach worker's telephone bill.

The personnel of this organization are some of the few concretely involved in community maintenance work. The center is staffed by a part-time mental health coordinator (the title for noncredentialed mental health workers) who supervises the center's hot lunch and social activities program. Her main contribution to maintaining confused elderly, however, is through telephone contact. She is responsible for telephoning between 15 and 25 mental health care referrals every day.

Mrs. Williams could never have been maintained in the community without her [senior citizen center director 1] help. She's the mainstay of our efforts. (psychiatric nurse 1, CSH)

I call her on the phone every day, and remind her to cash her Social Security check, things like that. She says, "I'm OK. I did all my errands." (senior citizen center director 1)

The community organizer is employed by the Religious Council to hustle the community for the seniors. From her point of view, elderly are confused as a result of political machinations, and political activism and community organization will solve their problems: "Some are eccentric-out, of sync with society. Theirs is a forced debilitation by deliberate exclusion.... They are politically confused by free rides and picnics" (community organizer). Her job is to capture general resources for seniors' use.

If she hears about something that might be useful, she's on the phone immediately. (psychiatric nurse 1, GST)

A center member became increasingly confused. Her neighbors forced her out of the building. We got $50 from the Religious Council, borrowed a neighbor's car, rented a U-Haul, and hired three kids from the OEO rent-a-kid project. We had her moved out in one day. (senior citizen director 3)

The geriatric social worker makes the rounds to all three senior citizen centers, the three neighborhood health centers, the Family Counselling Society, the Community Mental Health Center Geriatric Specialists, and city hall. Her job is to manage the movement of patients, make referrals to the neighborhood health centers, and take referrals from city hall. She was trained as a clinician to treat individuals, but in the community she is confronted with more pressing immediate needs.

You have schizophrenics and depressed old people who need therapy. They also have very concrete needs—money, housing, food—as well as complex personal problems. You can't separate one from the other. There aren't services to handle both, so you do it. (geriatric social worker)

Older people aren't interested in working with their problems. They aren't interested in changing their lives, but they do want someone to talk to. (geriatric social worker)

FAMILY COUNSELLING SOCIETY

For the caseworkers at the Family Counselling Society, confusion in the elderly is only a phase in a history of lifelong impairment. It is, after all, clients with this sort of impairment who could benefit most from the case worker skills.

The senile old people we deal with are people who have never coped well. It's not a matter of something happening in old age. (family counselor 1)

There are a lot of chronic noncopers, people inadequate throughout their lives. (family counselor 2)

These workers, like the geriatric social worker, experience conflict between their traditional roles and direct services. They have personally opted for doing the community maintenance work that no one else will do. But it is a problem for them to reconcile their professional identity with the work they think needs to be done.

The worse off the client is, the less likely he is to get help. No one wants the job of direct services. The professionals all want to be planners. That's fine, but who's going to do the work? Who do you send in when feces are smeared all over the house? You have to be tough. We do direct services even though we're not supposed to. We do it because that's what's needed. (family counselor 1)

I go out once a week and cash his checks for him. Now I'm trying to teach him budgeting. Of course he still needs counseling. (family counselor 1)

NURSING HOME ORGANIZER

A veterans' hospital in the metropolitan area has placed its discharged chronic patients in Claiborne nursing homes. A social worker from the hospital has initiated a unique community program in Claiborne. Nursing home residence is a prerequisite for membership. From the organizers' point of view, nursing home residents are more isolated than those who live alone. At a minimum, the organizers want to bring residents out of the home to see the community and meet new people. But pleasure is subordinated to business. At the group's semimonthly "business meetings" attended by residents from eight to ten nursing homes, members discussed patient advocacy inside the homes and means to air grievances publicly and assert their rights. At least, this is the organizers' framework for action.

Group work is more effective than one-to-one with this population. Our program gives them a chance to share common problems and learn from the experiences of others. It gives them a chance to complain. It makes them better self-advocates in the home. (nursing home organizer)

They learn about the community by actually being in it, traveling to different nursing homes, churches, and elderly housing projects. (nursing home organizer)

Because the vast majority of the membership is elderly and confused, a great deal of effort is involved in the more mundane aspects of organization, for instance, transportation. Ordering and loading and unloading a fleet of taxis is time consuming and too complex for residents to handle alone. The program depends on the nursing home recreation workers to find meeting places and to arrange transportation. Clearly, the success of the program depends on the leadership's ability to organize the nursing home workers as well as residents.

They may feel that the time it takes to arrange for transportation alone would be better spent with the patients. (nursing home organizer)

We spend the major portion of our time just transporting patients. We must do it all ourselves. No one else wants the job. (recreation worker, Autumn Nursing Home)

Getting residents to play their part is also problematic from the leaders' point of view:

People fall down; they get hurt; they sit silently at meetings. They don't have ideas, or the ones they do have don't work. (nursing home organizer)

Even the simplest elements of group process are complicated. An attempt to count the participants from each nursing home failed because too many members didn't know the name of their home. (observation)

On one occasion elaborate preparations were made for a luncheon. A representative from state government, and a panel of six residents were to speak on the problems of nursing home life. The speaker failed to appear, and the panel members had no complaints about nursing home care. One panel member urged greater reliance on God. A second extolled the virtues of self-help. "Try self-help as much as you can, and you'll be surprised." A third announced, "I enjoy nursing home life. We play games. I'm a fine whist player. It's fun." One member did complain about City Hospital, and was roundly criticized by vociferous City Hospital supporters in the audience. (observation)

In the last illustration above, the planned demonstration of complaints failed. Whether it was the dynamics of public complaint, group process captured by optimism, or an accurate representation of the membership's sentiments, the panel and audience did not play the part intended by the organizers. Nonetheless, large numbers of confused elderly (approximately 50 at a business meeting and 300 at the luncheon) have an unusual opportunity to leave nursing home premises. As recreation, the events are complete successes.

SHELTERED WORKSHOP FOR SENIORS

The senior workshop, which is located on the periphery of Claiborne, and funded by the Community Mental Health Center, offers its seniors "meaningful" occupational experiences:

Most programs today degrade the elderly, like arts and crafts and beano. As for hot lunches, who wants to eat the main meal of the day at one o'clock? And they have no choice about food. Elderly are asked to volunteer. We labor under the impression that we are a generous giving society. The only thing that matters is the buck. It's insulting to ask people to volunteer. But if Polaroid is willing to pay for this work the seniors are doing, then it must be meaningful. (CMHC sponsor)

Actually, the senior workshop depends on its parent organization, the Singer State Hospital workshop, to find enough work to occupy members. The senior workers make key chains, prepare pencil packages, and sew bras. "We call this the life saver. When there's nothing else to do, there's always the bras to fall back on" (senior worker). In spite of the center's close mental health affiliation, it only recently accepted an elderly ex-mental hospital patient: "The continuing care unit asked us to take one of their patients. We hassled. What will the rest think? We decided to try it because we didn't know what would happen" (CMHC sponsor). If the "psychiatrically enlightened" community stations are skeptical and reluctant to accept confused elderly, what can be expected from others that lack professional guidance?

WELFARE

In this state, the Welfare Department has been reorganized into two separate components: service and payment. A local service unit is situated on the fringe of Claiborne. The new welfare service unit manual claims the following services will be offered to the elderly: education, employment, chore services, foster care, medication, meals, homemaker, home management, health and mental health care, housing information and referrals, legal advice, and protective services. In reality, the service unit does two things: sends out taxi slips and approves homemaker services. If only a taxi slip is requested, the applicant is referred to the central office downtown.

The office is understaffed. There is supposed to be one intake worker, three generalists, and a resource mobilization person. Actually, there is a half-time resource mobilization person and a full-time generalist. The generalist has a case load of 215 elderly clients. Without adequate staff to perform services, the department is limited to handling bureaucratic formalities. Confused elderly come to them for help, and are turned away. The following is a summary of an encounter among an 82-year-old lady, her Salvation Army (abbreviated SA) companion, and the geriatric welfare worker:

> Lady: I've been waiting since 1959 for help from the city for housing. I've been goin' downhill since my husband died, and I've been all over since then looking for help.
>
> SA: She's got to find somewhere else to live. There's no bathroom. She can't prepare food. She only gets $105 a month, and she has to pay $65 of that for rent.
>
> Lady: When I move, I want to be near a laundry. And I'd like to move in the springtime.
>
> Welfare: Well, you apply for housing at the downtown office.
>
> SA: We waited all day yesterday at some welfare office, and they sent us here. They said she'd get a social worker, someone to help her with these things.
>
> Welfare: Well, we only do home care and taxi slips.
>
> SA: Why did they send us here? Doesn't she have a social worker?
>
> Welfare: I can tell you where to go for housing.
>
> SA: What about money? Can she get any more money?
>
> Welfare: We don't have anything to do with payments.

In the office conversation after the lady and her companion departed, the workers acknowledged the agency's inadequacy:

> We get this kind of confused old lady in here two or three times a week. Usually they come with a relative. It's too bad you can't do something to help someone like that. But we've never been able to do anything for them. People just don't want one-to-one contact. It's hard to find someone to take on these cases. (supervisor)

NEIGHBORHOOD HEALTH CENTER

Confused elderly who go to the neighborhood health clinic are seen in the medical clinic for physical ailments. The mental health clinic is unwilling to treat them.

> Some are so disorganized—what meaning can life have? They might as well die. I know that sounds cruel but.... Our services are needed for more severe, more complex personality problems. (psychiatric nurse, mental health clinic)

Lady: Maybe I should find someone to take care of the cats, and get it over with.
Counselor: Listen, if you're not feeling too good about yourself, you should go see the psychiatrist at the clinic.
Lady: I've already been there. He says there's nothing he can do for me.

The mental health workers are accused of having a bad attitude by the community maintenance workers:

They are pessimistic about treating old people. They make assumptions about diagnostic stability. They believe senility is irreversible, and there's nothing you can do about it. They don't treat old people. It's mostly a matter of trying to change their attitude. (geriatric social worker)

The mental health workers are conventional in their diagnostic judgments and rely on standardized measures of senility. The health care workers are skeptical of the standardized mental status exam and describe alternative indicators of confusion. Their indicators focus more on competence in meeting daily needs than on mental skills.

I end up talking in circles every time I try to think of characteristics of senility. Every time I think of a characteristic, I can think of an alternative explanation. (nurse, health clinic)

I hate the mental status exam. I never use it. It's so insulting. Whenever I have to use it, I always preface it with, "Now I'm going to ask you a lot of silly questions to test your memory." (nurse, health clinic)

This guy reads Latvian newspapers so he may not know who the president is. Does that mean he's senile? (nurse, health clinic)

In place of standardized measurements, they employ these indicators of confusion:

... when they start to have problems with their money, like refusing to pay their bills (community worker). ... when they don't understand the instructions I give them for a physical exam (nurse, health clinic). ... when they seem well-motivated, but just don't do things like take medicines or keep appointments (nurse, health clinic). ... when they can't tell me what they did today (nurse, health clinic).

In this setting it is only the community workers and medical nurses who have responsibility for handling the confused elderly. Their perspective emphasizes observation of personal and health maintenance ability.

PRIVATE PHYSICIANS

Private physicians define confusion as a medical problem, so they do not consult psychiatric specialists. Mental health workers are considered to be less competent at diagnosing a medical problem.

> I never use Central State Hospital for my senile patients. (private physician 3)

> Central State Hospital is not much of a resource for determining the mental status of a confused elderly person. If I wanted to find the medical grounds for reversible illness, they'd be a poor choice. (private physician 2)

The physicians are pessimistic about improvement in elderly, and therefore see their job in terms of medical management and the mobilization of community resources:

> If all the physical tests come up negative, we tell the family there's nothing we can do except place him. (private physician 2)

> The first thing to do is try medicines, the vasodilators. I try a patient on one or two of them. They might appear to help, and occasionally a patient does improve, but they usually don't do any good. (private physician 3)

> There's no useful medical treatment for senility. (private physician 2)

The primary role of the private physician is house doctor for the nursing homes. In the role of house doctor, the point of view remains the same, but the physician encourages the participation of mental health specialists in managing behavior problems. Medication and discharge are the issues that bring them together. Yet the house doctors and the mental health specialists have conflicting ideas, so their relationship is often antagonistic:

> Most of them who come from the hospital are in another world. Will medication control? That's the only question. With the new pills today almost all of them can be managed. Those who can't should go to Central State Hospital. They have facilities and specialized staff to work with these problems. (private physician 1)

Medicating the nursing home patient has been described as a compromise among the principal actors—the head nurse, the house doctor, and the psychiatric consultant. The negotiations between the house doctor and the consultant are complex and sensitive. They include mutual accusations of ignorance, incompetence, and misuse of medication. The basic complaint of the psychiatric consultant is that nursing home doctors underuse tranquilizers because they are ignorant of their "proper" use and are afraid of them:

> Nursing home physicians are kind of out of touch. They're generally old, and not exactly in the forefront of medical practice. They probably never were. They tend to be cautious and conservative. (psychiatric resident 2, CSH)

> They tend to underuse tranquilizers. They don't prescribe accurately. They aren't aware of interactions and side effects. (psychiatrist, GST)

House doctors, on the other hand, accuse psychiatrists of "snowing" patients and experimenting with medication:

> They use massive doses of drugs. If I order 25 mg., they'd order 200. I always use the least, not the most. I'm not going to make zombies out of my patients. (private physician 1)

> They experiment with medications. They use combinations of two or more drugs, and who knows what happens inside the body when all those chemicals interact. (private physician 2)

REDEFINED ROLES AND TEMPERED ASSESSMENT

For most community managers, community work involves carrying out the functions of their particular agency in a manner consistent with their own professional training. Community maintenance work rarely falls within the self-defined role of agencies or professionals. For example, one characteristic of the work is the need for daily contact with the individual. Community workers who take on maintenance duties consider it to be the overriding factor in maintaining a person in the community: "I've learned to make daily visits immediately, then taper off. They never get to recognize you if you don't. Once a week isn't often enough" (geriatric social worker). However, institutional employees (for example at Central State Hospital) who do community work consider the time spent in street transit to be wasteful. They think community visits once or twice a week are "frequent." They do not make daily telephone contacts with community residents since that is a job for nonprofessionals.

Most professionals define maintenance work as uncomplicated, simple-minded work that anyone with a little training can do. Professionals consider themselves to be overqualified for such work, and believe they can more effectively use their skills to consult with other managers, train nonprofessionals, and mobilize resources (Caro 1974). In essence, community maintenance is, from the specialists' point of view, "dirty work." Various community agents provided the following illustrations:

... taking out the trash. ... negotiating with the landlord who wanted our client out. ... I call her on the phone every single day. ... moving furniture. ... going to her home to find her housing application. ... making arrangements to have her house defleaed. ... taking her shopping.

There are a few professionals who do the dirty work in spite of being "overqualified" because they cannot find anyone else to do it. Their presence on the street and in private residences has made them vulnerable to situations they cannot avoid. Yet their professional identity is at stake in reconciling the disparity between their offer of psychological relief, personal growth, and emotional mastery and the confused elderly's need for concrete, pragmatic help (Nadler 1973; Mayadas and Hink 1974). The work is described as more frustrating than rewarding. They look forward to being released from "front-line" obligations by changing jobs or by occupational advancement.

> The problem with this job is that you must deal with the concrete as well as personal problems of your client. You must figure out if there's enough money to pay the rent. You must fill out welfare and housing applications for them. But you also have schizophrenics who need therapeutic counseling. Which do you undertake? Even if you wanted to, you can't separate one from the other. And if you could, there aren't the service people to handle it. (geriatric social worker)

In addition to this redefinition of their jobs, doing dirty work in the community leads professionals to temper their diagnosis of confusion, senility, and organic brain disease. They see nonconventional behavior as survival strategies:

> She had telephone wire wrapped all around the door. Was it confusion or reasonable precaution? (social worker, PH)

> She's definitely senile. It's hardening of the arteries, depression, and paranoia. She doesn't answer the door. But she's very hard of hearing, and no one ever rings the doorbell, so it's no wonder. (geriatric social worker)

These workers rely less on standardized psychiatric diagnosis, and in some cases are hostile to its use:

> Senility is diagnostically very hard to pinpoint. (family counselor 1)

> I never use the mental status exam. It's demeaning. (nurse, NHC)

> The old person may be considered senile, but they know where their money is, and when the welfare check comes in. (nurse, NHC)

Certain confused behaviors, generally accepted as symptoms of senility, are redefined as personal problems in daily management.

CONCLUSIONS

The community care concept is viable if local servicing stations are willing to do long-term maintenance work with confused elderly. Maintenance needs, however, can become extremely complicated and stations are not always willing to cooperate. Claiborne social agents cover the gamut from total disavowal to complete engrossment in the confused elderly's daily problems. Individually, stations and agents project points of view that explain their "appropriate" dissociation from the dirty work. It is the exceptions—nursing home organizer, geriatric social worker, community organizer, and family counselor—who prove the general rule. For the others, encounters with confused elderly are brief, even for the private physician who may be tranquilizing confused nursing home residents.

5

THE NURSING HOME

Social scientists agree that the rapid growth of the nursing home industry has provided for the elderly a "community" alternative to the state mental hospital. By 1963, the nursing home industry had become a resource of care for the elderly with a psychiatric label second only to state and county mental hospitals. By 1967, more elderly with psychiatric diagnoses were in nursing homes than all other psychiatric inpatient facilities (Redick, Kramer and Taube 1973).

THE HOUSE AND ITS STAFF

The Court Nursing Home, the major resource for nursing home data, is one of the eight homes in the Claiborne area owned by a large corporation operating in the state. In terms of physical structure, location, and staff-resident ratio, it is typical of the level three nursing homes. The Court Nursing Home is a renovated wood frame house with 41 beds. There are 20 female residents on the main floor, 21 male residents upstairs. Each bedroom has from three to six beds. A dayroom on the main floor accommodates a maximum of 20 people. There are always six or seven ladies in the room with the television set turned on. Upstairs, the men congregate in the hallway by another television set, and any social activity takes place in this area. The bedrooms are neat and orderly. All the bedspreads and matching drapes are in bright floral patterns.

The lobby is the center of business and social activity for the home. Unlike many homes, there are no physical barriers between the main entrance and the resident population. Consequently, residents mill around the doorway and the nurses' station. The lobby, like the dayroom, belongs to the women. Men are rarely seen.

In the 12 years the nurse administrator (also titled head nurse) has worked at Court, there have been three different owners. The head nurse and the evening and night supervisors are LPNs. The home is otherwise staffed with nursing aides and attendants. Three of the aids have worked in the home for more than five years.

Nursing homes are required to have personnel responsible for social activities, either a social worker, recreational worker, or activities director. These workers are at the bottom of the staff hierarchy, as managing social and recreational events is not respected as serious work.

> Nurses don't take us seriously. We get a very small salary and no respect. They think we're just having a good time with the patients. (recreational worker, Bank)

> The nursing home is required to have social services, but I'm not sure they really want us. (activities director, Holst)

The ratio of recreational workers to residents varies among the homes, but in general workers are scarce.

> There's one activities director for two homes. One home has 100 patients-the other, between 50 and 75. We have a therapy room with all kinds of materials, but it's never open. There's no one to teach anyone how to do anything. It just isn't used. (resident, Majestic)

For these reasons, these workers have a small impact on the social quality of life inside the home.

Other ancillary staff to the home, the cooks and caretakers, might become involved with patients, depending on their outlook and the home regulations.

> I run errands for them—buy food, candy, cigarettes. No harm done in bein' decent. God forbid I should ever end up like that. (retired nursing home caretaker)

> In the home where I work, they don't want you to be too friendly with the patients. They don't want you to visit with them even if it's on your own time. (cook, Walden)

The head nurse is the most important figure in the nursing home. She is frequently identified as the basic determinant of the home's approach to care.

> Good homes become bad ones, and bad ones become good. It changes with the administrator. (continuing care nurse 1, CH)

> The head nurse has to be a good businesswoman as well as nurse. It's up to
> her to keep the doors open. (head nurse, Holst)

She has extensive control over the resident's lives; residents will enter and leave
the home on her orders. Even the confused recognized her power. For example, as Mary (a discharged mental hospital patient) talked with me, she constantly listened to the night supervisor. She said, "I've done my time and I've
learned to keep track of her." On several occasions the head nurse "joked"
with patients about evicting them.

> [The head nurse pretended she wanted to take a dime from an elderly lady.
> When the lady was encouraged by an aide to refuse, everyone laughed.] Head
> nurse (in a teasing fashion): If you don't give it to me, I'm gonna put you
> out on the street. (Court)

The nurse's intent was to be jovial and lighthearted, and thereby show her
rapport with the residents. The resident, however, was unnerved by the joking
and pleaded, "Don't do that. I've no place to go." (Helen, Court).

Though her style may be intimidating to the residents, she is their advocate, arbitrator, and protector. When a resident timidly approached the head
nurse about a continuing linen problem, the nurse was annoyed that the
resident had waited so long to acknowledge her authority: "Why didn't you
come to me before? You have a problem, you know who to see to get action"
(head nurse, Holst).

When conflicts arise that cannot be settled on the spot, the staff will "let
her settle it when she comes in tommorrow." Only she has the last word. In
one case, an elderly lady was convinced that she would be evicted, and the head
nurse declared: "Now cut that out, Carol. No one can put you out on the street
but me, and I ain't gonna do it" (Court). The head nurse at Court takes on
outsiders on the residents' behalf. When the local branch of the public library
wouldn't admit her residents to a movie because the community people did not
want to mingle with them, she complained to City Hall, and the library movies
were reintegrated. When the neighbors called the police because the residents'
outdoor party was too loud, she refused to back down, and the party went on.

The head nurse's authority is not absolute. She is constrained by financial,
social, and legal checks on the home's operation. The nurse administrator, like
the rest of the staff, is an employee. Nursing homes are often criticized for
being understaffed and ill-equipped, but the head nurse does not control the
number of house staff, access to equipment and supplies, or even the residents'
daily menu. While the owners guard the profit margin, she must meet her
residents' daily needs with the resources available. Ownership and management are largely separate worlds in the multihome corporation.

Nursing homes must also be concerned with their appearance in the community. This sometimes presents special problems with the confused. The staff is aware that some of the residents on the street do not reflect a favorable impression of the home, but these ill-clad and ill-mannered residents refuse to cooperate. If they do not want to lock up residents, the situation must be endured. "She won't comb her hair. She won't wash. She goes out in the cold with sneakers and a sweater. Then the neighbors call and give us a hard time. She really puts you over the barrel when she does that" (staff nurse, Bank).

Neighbors are skeptical and critical of the homes. Though they rarely go inside, they do see patients outside, and have opinions about life inside:

> The nursing home has a "who the fuck are you" attitude. They are very hostile over there. The people look so lonely. It'd be nice to have more community involvement but the staff is so intimidating. (neighbor 1)

> Sometimes we hear screams in the middle of the night. We don't know if we should call. It would probably be too late to intervene, and we're afraid of causing reprisals against a patient. (neighbor 2)

> We saw the attendant bait him and pull his hair, until the old man tried to kick him. We hollered out the window, and told the man to cut it out. (neighbor 3)

The home is subject to frequent inspection by the ownership, insurance companies, the department of public health, and placement personnel from the hospitals. Five different certificates of accreditation and licenses hang on the lobby wall. It even has a restaurant license. The staff complains that overinspection and overregulation are deleterious to the residents' comfort and well-being as well as disruptive to their own jobs:

> It's against the rules to have patients working in the kitchen, but I let Ella do it because she likes it so much. On Sunday the kitchen staff wouldn't let her. She didn't like that, so she left. She was gone for two days, and finally came back in a cab. (head nurse, Court)

> I'm trying to break the routine of getting patients out of bed, and having their beds made by a certain time. Who are we to tell them they can't sleep late if they want? But if visitors and inspectors come and see things looking disorderly, then we have problems. The regulations say the beds are supposed to be made every day. (head nurse, Court)

> It's inspection time here so we had to make a few extra preparations, like going around and taking the food out of patients' drawers. It's not allowed. (recreation worker, Autumn)

CONFUSION IN THE VERNACULAR

Frequently the admitting diagnosis to a nursing home includes terms like "chronic brain" syndrome, "senile psychosis," or "organic brain" syndrome (Saul and Saul 1974). There is, however, a decline in the use and importance of such terms once the elderly person is in the home. In some cases, supervisors actively lobby against their use.

> I don't believe in senility. I don't use the word, and I don't want the staff to use the word. (administrator, Thompson Nursing Home Corporation)

> We don't use the words like senility or demented. We don't talk about mental illness. (head nurse, Holst)

Mental health workers who lead patient groups in nursing homes describe the staff as antagonistic toward the idea of psychiatric treatment.

> They accused us of doing psychotherapy, and said they didn't want any of that. (group leader, CSH)

> The home insisted on describing our group as a coffee-luncheon. They didn't even want the word "therapy" used. (group leader, CSH)

The psychiatric terminology is replaced with vernacular expressions:

> . . . She's cracked, too bad (staff nurse 1, Court). . . . something is the matter with his squash (head nurse, Holst). . . . it's just like being a vegetable (activities director, Holst). . . . They're deficient in certain chemicals (administrator, Clover). . . . some of them are "way out," (activities director, Autumn). . . . most of them are already in another world (house doctor, Court). . . . they're just out in the backyard, and there ain't no back door (staff nurse 1, Court).

The ideology of psychiatric treatment is replaced by humanistic rhetoric.

> Tender loving care is what they get here. (administrator, Thompson Nursing Home Corporation)

> You go by the Golden Rule, and it will come out alright in the end. (staff nurse 1, Court)

> What you do with elderly is called empathy. We try to put ourselves in their place, get into their world. (staff nurse 1, Court)

In the absence of specific conflict, the nursing home staff's attitude is generally benevolent. Overt hostility or notions of futility are not a conspicuous part of their thinking. The resident is a "patient" and deserves special consideration:

If you take the time you can understand even a babbler. (head nurse, Court)

A lot of times they just can't coordinate their hands and minds. (night supervisor, Court)

The residents are also recognized as a cooperative and useful participants in the home. They help make beds, clean, run errands, etc. (Although homes are sometimes accused of exploiting residents to do maintenance work in the house, the residents were anxious to help or at least willing to volunteer.)

The patients are helpful. If someone falls, they want to help pick them up. But you take Patty—she tries to lift them up by their feet. (staff nurse 1, Court)

The patients are helpful—they like to clean up. Some have their own job. One lady sweeps and dusts the TV room. If anyone else does it, she gets upset. One lady like to wash trays, another runs errands, and one works in the kitchen. (head nurse, Court)

The confused elderly women who mingle in the lobby make still another contribution to the home, one not acknowledged by the staff. These women act as buffers between staff and residents in times of conflict. In the following illustration, two of the home's most confused ladies, Blondie and Patty, who rarely utter an intelligible phrase, tried to calm the actors after this hostile exchange:

Nurse: Get back in your room?
Lady: Shut up! Mind your own business!
Nurse: It is my business! I have to take care of you. You'll fall down. It's for your own good that you have to stay in your room.
Blondie [to the lady]: Why don't you go back to your room?
Patty [to the nurse]: It's O.K., she don't mean nothin' by it.

MEETING DAILY NEEDS

The average citizen, as well as the social scientist and the politician, has a sense of the nursing home problem. The elderly are terrified by the thought of spending their last days in a home. Being in a nursing home is equated with decline and death. Residents feel abandoned, and families resign themselves to the necessity of placement (Suster 1971). The news media regularly publish the discovery of another nursing home scandal. Departments of public health and welfare crack down on offenders. Senate subcommittees and local politicians investigate. Corporate owners are accused of gouging out huge profits and of inadequately providing for residents (Mendelson 1975; Anderson 1974). The nursing home is the only station faced with the task of long-term daily management for large numbers of confused elderly. They have replaced the mental hospital as the station of last resort. As such, they are subject to the criticisms once applied to the hospital, that the institution's needs for economy and efficiency are incompatible with individuals' needs for freedom, privacy, and private property.* Institutional efficiency and order determine the methods of preparation and service of meals, bathing and toileting, and even group laundering and indiscriminate redistribution of personal clothing. Regulations subdue spontaneity and self-expression, and residents are depersonalized and desocialized.

The polarity of institutional and individual interests is well illustrated in an incident reported by the chef at the Main Street luncheonette:

> He went back to the state hospital. They got rid of him in a hurry because he took a whack at a nurse. He wrote me a letter explaining what happened. He woke up in the middle of the night and asked for some orange juice. They refused, and he got angry. They told him it's against regulations, but they could have given him some on the 'QT'. The whole scene would've been avoided and he wouldn't have been shipped out.

A point of view popular with social scientists is expressed in the following assessment of the problem:

> ... their procedures create excessive disability, transforming the resident into a more medically dependent person whose now more simplified needs can be met in a highly structured and less personalized environment. Do not nursing homes, in common with all institutions, create the very type of patients, inmate or resident that it wants as well as needs to justify its very existence? (Tobin 1974)

They recommend that the nursing homes should:

> ... be modelled more on normal life roles, fostering independence, social contacts, and meaningful activities. (Gottesman 1974)

---

*It is my impression that these criticisms are made even more vigorously of the nursing home because of its greater social visibility to neighbors and family, and because it lacks the appearance of professional affiliation that mental hospitals claimed with respect to psychiatry. Whether or not the nursing home is better or worse than the mental hospital as an institutional environment is an issue of popular debate. I touch on this question in the summary of the paper.

... [facilitate] environments characterized by high degrees of autonomy fostering, personalization of patients, community integration. (Lieberman 1974)

The simple dichotomy between the patients' needs and the institution's needs is the common professional explanation for the nursing homes' problems. The staff, however, does not accept this, because they are faced with complexities of management that this explanation does not take into account. Their general framework for action could be constructed as follows:

Quality care is not easy to define. If we force an unstable walker to stay in bed, we're too hospital oriented and overprotective. If that person falls, breaks a hip, goes to the hospital, gets pneumonia, and dies on the orthopedic ward, then we feel guilty and neglectful. If we let out a potential wanderer, and she gets lost or hurt or mugged, then we were wrong, but the only alternative may be to restrain her. We have to do what we think is best for the patient. Our choices are limited by the resources available, and sometimes there just is no right answer. The basic problem is not that patients must conform to our routine, but that all kinds of people must learn to live together under one roof. We have blacks and whites, the loud and the quiet, Jews and Christians, the timid and the hostile, the loners and the gregarious, the normal and senile. In a communal setting, everyone has to make compromises. Our job is to protect the interests of everyone.

Conviviality

Spontaneous conviviality among patients within a nursing home is rare because of a repressive social environment and individual incapacity. One study of nursing homes concluded that staff regards conversations among patients as silly and meaningless. Only aides and nurses have the power of speech and are capable of demanding a response from another staff person (Stannard 1973). Another study reported that patient conversation is considered to be potentially disruptive, and is discouraged (Stotsky 1970). Every day, Alice sits on her bed in her room, and across the hall, Katie sits in a chair behind her door. They identify each other as friends. On outings they like to travel and eat together. They have similar Irish backgrounds. Both have physical disabilities, but ambulate. Yet they do not cross the hallway to visit one another. Their self-imposed isolation seems to be a response to conversational norms.

There are extreme isolates totally removed from any conviviality. They sit in the same spot every day without speaking to anyone or being spoken to. Those who sit in a chair next to their bed, eat from a portable tray attached to their chair, and use a portable toilet next to the chair have a total life limited to several inches. There is no room for socializing:

> You go in there, and you'll see them. Some of them no one ever comes near. (retired nursing home caretaker)
>
> I like to have someone to talk to once in awhile. It's a killer. (Ed, 94-year-old resident, Court)

In most cases these total isolates do not respond immediately to conversational overtures. Either they cannot or prefer not to speak. When they do speak, they are difficult to understand because of their disjointed, apparently incoherent choice of words. Under these circumstances, casual spontaneous conversation is very improbable. As long as these patients do not complain or disturb, their isolation goes uninterrupted.

There are exceptions to the pattern of daily isolation, usually among the women. The most gregarious and socially aggressive manage to create convivial opportunities.

> Nellie gets all dressed up when her boyfriend is coming. If he doesn't show up, she goes out looking for him. Yesterday she found him in a bar with another woman, and claims she slapped both of them. I believe it too. (head nurse, Court)
>
> We had one couple that wanted to get married. We cleared it with the administration. At the last minute she caught him cheating on her, and backed out of the wedding. (head nurse, Court)

Recreation and Remotivation

The nursing homes' answer to the lack of conviviality is to extend their residents' social lives with organized recreational activities. Wednesday afternoon barbeque, beano (a substitute for bingo, and played in an identical manner), arts and crafts, and shopping on Main Street are the usual events. An annual outing to the amusement park, the mayor's picnic, the cocktail party, and the city's summer program with sing-a-longs for seniors are special events. In addition, a new technique of therapeutic recreation, called remotivation therapy, has found its way into several nursing homes in Claiborne.

The staff is convinced that participation in these events is good for residents and that residents should take advantage of the opportunities. It can be difficult to find willing participants, however. Residents complained that it was too much work to move the chairs outdoors for the barbeque. They preferred to eat indoors. Some refuse to play beano: "Who wants to play for candy and dimes? That's kids' stuff" (Mary, Court). They complained about being coerced into going to the amusement park:

I didn't want to go. It wasn't good for me. The ride was too long, and I got too tired. And I had to pay $3.40 for the bus. I don't know if I can afford it. (Katie, Court)

Lizzie (resident): I'm very ill. I want to go home.
Head nurse: This is the first time you've been out since you came to the Court. You always pretend to be sick. This is your day, so enjoy yourself. Come over and sit in this easy chair. Are you going to dance?
Lizzie: I can't even hold up my head. I was sick last night.

Nursing homes face the dilemma of enforcing participation against the residents' will or accepting refusals and tolerating decisions that contradict their definitions of the patients' best interests. The only residents who actually went on the roller coaster and other freak rides were those too confused to protest.

Recreation worker (Court): I don't force them to go on trips.
Head nurse: Well, I do, or they come back to you next day saying, "You didn't want me to go; you didn't make me." If they go, they enjoy themselves. If they stay home, they just sit in the TV room. It's good for them to go whether they want to or not.

Even the simplest of structured recreational activities is complicated when confused residents are included. For example, playing beano becomes an exercise in managing group confusion. (In some homes, beano is only open to those who can play on their own.) The recreational worker calls out numbers, and another worker or aide scans the cards of the residents who are unable to play without assistance. When appropriate, the aide holds a finger over the proper box until the dependent player covers it with a marker. In essence, the staff plays the card, but, with assistance, the dependent players are as likely to win as their self-sufficient counterparts. Everyone has a sense of winning. Even those most detached from the mechanics of the game are pleased when someone explains to them that they won. The prize is a dime or choice of candy bar. At the end of a game, there are several residents who must be instructed to clear their cards so that a new game can begin.

Unlike recreational activities, remotivation therapy claims a theoretical rationale and offers a specific format of practice. Remotivation therapy is not part of the medical or mental health operations. In fact, its ideology is specifically nonpsychiatric:

... a simple technique to reach the unwounded parts of the patient's personality. Most of these patients have some brain damage. We are working with the undamaged part of the brain. (remotivation therapist, Autumn)

... topics are designed to focus on the nonpathological interests. (Toepfer 1974)

The concept is an adaptation of the behavior modification model to the nursing home setting, where "abnormal behavior" is thought to be frequently rewarded. This program rewards "normal behavior" (Toepfer 1974). Anyone can be trained to do remotivation therapy. Special training programs train remotivation therapists, and they, in turn, train the nonprofessional nursing home staff. Anyone can benefit. "This is a program for the needs of every patient except the dying and the comatose" (remotivation therapist, Autumn).

A remotivation session is expected to follow the following pattern (from Toepfer 1974; remotivation therapist, Autumn):

1. Climate of acceptance; make a positive comment to reward each individual for coming
2. Bridge to reality; read a rhythmical poem or article—this is a source of stimulation (verbal and social); put patients in touch with reality through affective poetry
3. Nonpathological topics (topics relating to illness or family relations and controversial subjects such as religion or prejudice are avoided); topic selected to share the world we live in
4. Patient relates his own life experiences to the topic
5. Climate of appreciation; leader expresses personal pleasure in working with the group

Putting the program into practice at the Autumn House proved complex. An elaborate planned-in-advance program requires a deliberate, calculated selection process. The selection process used for beano games, going from room to room and canvassing residents, is not adequate. Patients must be found who are confused but not too confused, who need to be remotivated but can at least respond to questions, who are a little withdrawn but communicative. It is important not to include too many "distracting" patients (anyone who would make a scene).

"Consistency of approach is the key to rehabilitation of confused patients," according to the therapist's manual. A program of constant, 24-hour reorientation proposed in the manual calls for a half-hour of intensive classroom orientation every day, and outside the classroom the staff is "to carry on the conversation, to get everyone on the ward talking about the classroom topic." Unfortunately, in the remotivation program at Autumn, the therapist came only once a week for two hours. Daily sessions were impossible. Further-more, only three of the nursing home staff were involved, and even they were unwilling to try to keep the topic alive for a whole week.*

While these remotivation sessions were intended for the benefit of the patients, they were also training sessions for the nursing home attendants. The therapist took the position that "If the attendants don't come, it isn't worth doing." In other words, helping the residents was, by itself, an insufficient rationale for the program's existence. Two attendants and the recreational worker had been assigned by the nursing home to attend the meetings. By the third week, the attendants openly opposed their continued participation.

> Trainee 1: Do we have to come?
> Therapist: Yes, I would like you to.
> Trainee 2: [to the other]: I'm not coming any more. As long as I don't have anything better to do than play, I might as well play upstairs with the patients.

The attendants were insulted rather than honored that they had been chosen to participate. They believed that they got along fine with patients, and did not need this training. In addition, they had their usual work to complete on the floor. Attending sessions only made their jobs more difficult; they had just as much work, but less time. The therapist saw the developing situation like this: "I thought this was a cooperative place, but they don't want to be bothered. The administration isn't really interested. They won't push the staff."

Given the unsuccessful selection process, the infrequency of the sessions, the lack of enthusiasm by staff for a program they don't believe in, the thera-pist's own unwillingness to continue solely for the sake of the residents, it is not obvious that the residents benefited from the sessions. The principle was not implemented in this setting, and therefore its usefulness was not tested.

Liberty and Protective Custody

Loss of personal freedom appears in almost every daily function inside the home. Restrictions on the residents' freedom to move freely inside the home and to enter and leave the home at will is the major problem. The balance between protective custody, as perceived by the staff, and personal liberty, as perceived by residents, is the most controversial of the daily management

---

*The first topic discussed was cats. The staff thought the subject was banal, and two of them later admitted to an active dislike of cats. They even disliked hearing the therapist talk about them.

encounters. Placement organizations report that wanderers are some of the most difficult patients to place; nursing homes refuse to accept them. (A wanderer is any resident who either runs away from the home or gets lost outside and needs assistance getting back.) From the residents' point of view, the loss of freedom is the most aggravating of the violations to personal integrity:

> I find it very difficult to be in a place like this. In someways it's like a prison, only the prisoners have done nothing to deserve being in jail. God help those who end up in a real prison. (Katie, Court)

> [An elderly gentleman on the orthopedic ward at City Hospital was barely able to talk]
> Nurse: Do you like the nursing home?
> Man: No.
> Nurse: Why not?
> Man: [garbled answer]
> Nurse: I can't understand what you say.
> Man: [with clenched fist and clear voice]: Because they took away my freedom!

Freedom of mobility is restricted when the staff is afraid a resident will fall, get lost, or otherwise endanger themselves.

> We're sometimes too soft and oversympathetic. She fell because people thought she could walk. We wanted to give her a chance. (staff nurse 1, Court)

> I don't let her out on Friday afternoon because I know she's goin' drinking, then you never know what will happen. (head nurse, Court)

> There are only three patients in the home who can walk away without getting lost. (staff nurse, Court)

The nursing home staff thinks wandering is a consequence of mental confusion. Outsiders (police, neighbors) attribute it to boredom in the home, restlessness, or looking for fun and adventure. When Blondie left and was returned several hours later by the police, she grinned and raised her eyebrows when asked about the policemen. It seemed she had a good time. Wanderers are poor informants of their own activities. Blondie could not provide a coherent account of her outing. When Ella returned after a two-day absence, the head nurse (Court) tried in vain to reconstruct the event.

> Head nurse: You tell me where you went!
> Ella: I don't remember where I went or what I did.

Head nurse: Did you have a drink?
Ella: I might have. Drink's the only thing that takes away my memory.
Head nurse: Did you go to a movie?
Ella: I might have. I love movie pictures.
Head nurse: You've got a nice tan so I know you've been outside.
Ella: Well, I like to walk.

Nursing home personnel attempt to restrain potential wanderers. Medical orders are used for this purpose:

If it's written in the medical orders "no outside privileges," then it's illegal for us to let them out. If they do sneak away, there's nothing we can do about it. We aren't legally responsible. Someone without outside privileges can go out with supervision or on a group bus or trip. (head nurse, Court)

The orders are on a form sheet that the nursing home administrator usually fills out, since the placement institution does not. It is then signed by the house physician who is assigned to the patient. In other words, the right to go outdoors is at the discretion of the head nurse who must make her decision on little or no information. The staff also impresses on the returnee of the danger of his or her action:

Head nurse (Court): This is the third time you've done it. It's dangerous out on the street. Once the police brought you back when they found you wandering the streets in the middle of the night. Another time you got drunk, and the police took you to the hospital. What happened to your pocketbook?
Ella: I don't know. I must have had it with me.
Head Nurse: You had at least $30 plus your kitchen earnings. I can't do anything about your money. If you were in any of those bars near the station, you probably lost it there. Somebody probably put a mickey in your drink. I understand they're good about that when they see you've got money.

The following physical adjustments make wandering difficult or impossible:

One way nursing homes deal with wanderers is to take away their shoes and give them slippers. It may help, and it's a lot better than tying them to a chair. (nurse practitioner 1, CH)

Fred is a wanderer. Give him his pants and he's gone. (staff nurse 2, Court)

If you don't get back to your room, you're gonna be tied to a chair. (night supervisor, Court)

Tying down a resident is an unpleasant job, but accepted with equanimity:

The Court staff had reason to believe that a new admission might try to run away. While I was talking with the new admission, two nurses entered the room, apologized for the interruption, unfolded a bed sheet, stretched it out and spun it in the air until it was tightly wound. They tied the resident to the steel frame bedpost with this sheet, and fixed it in a large bulky knot behind his back so he couldn't reach it. Of course he couldn't lean back in his chair either. (observation)

When the wanderer is lost or runs away, the staff is faced with the problem of getting the resident back. Some never come back; some are returned by police; some are apprehended in flight.

Some of them go the same way everytime. They're not too hard to find. For instance, we had one lady who was just like lightning, she was so fast. She went to the housing project every time, so I'd jump in my car, drive over there, and bring her back. (head nurse, Court)

Once she was gone overnight. No one could find her. Then in the morning we got a call to go to this apartment building. When I got there, she tried to close the door on me. She made a scene, but I took her out anyway. She didn't have any clothes on, and there wasn't anyone around, so I figured she wasn't doing very well outside. Even if she didn't want to go, she'd be better off at the home. (head nurse, Court)

Helen, a resident at Autumn, announced that she was leaving, packed a small handbag, and walked out the door unnoticed. Her departure was spotted by the head nurse of the home next door and inquired at Autumn. An aide was sent to retrieve Helen, who adamantly refused to return. The aided coaxed, "You didn't tell anyone good-bye. You look tired. Come back and rest. You're not properly dressed. You're going to miss the party this afternoon." Helen did not give in, and was finally returned by the police. Within half an hour she made it out the door again, and was returned by a more forceful aide. A third attempt to get out was once again halted by the neighboring nursing home. Helen gave up, and returned to her room. (observation)

Property

Erving Goffman (1959) pointed out the conflict between institutional efficiency and the presence of personal possessions. Most of the elderly's personal possessions are lost in the transition from community resident to nursing home resident:

. . . the old are denied most segments—if not all—of their previous life style. Furniture, therefore, even when inadequately hospital-designed, is used by the facility for the aged often times more inadequately than their original, less than perfect intent. (Kaplan 1974)

Those possessions that do survive are out of place. A story apparently popular among professionals outside the home documents this (I read or heard a similar story on several occasions): "I wanted to put a picture of her children on the dresser, but the aide insisted I put it in the drawer. She didn't want it on top where she had to dust." (continuing care worker 2, CSH).

Clothing is the one form of property that occasionally survives the transition into the home, but keeping track of it is a problem.

> When I first came here I had a fur coat and a beautiful sweater. When I asked the head nurse what became of them, she said I was mistaken, that I never had a fur coat. But I know I had it. I don't say she was lying, but she probably thought I was mental, and making it up. (Katie, Court)

Residents acquire new clothing from a traveling salesman who serves the corporation homes. The head nurse encourages residents to select their clothes from his stock. Some of them complain that his prices are too high, and the choice too limited.

> Now look at it. They bought me these shoes and they look like bookends. Isn't that terrible. And I had to pay $14.95. (Katie, Court)

> He is a little expensive. (recreational worker, Court)

New clothes may become common property in the group laundry: "Even if you get new clothes they go into the laundry unmarked, and you never get them back" (Katie, Court). Often residents contest the owership of dresses and sweaters. If the item is unlabeled, the staff has to decide who wore it last. Other residents refuse to wear new clothes when they get them: "She has all the new clothes she wants, but she won't wear them. We hide all her old clothes in the laundry room so she'll wear the new ones." (Head nurse, Court). Some of the residents arrive with no clothing at all, and no money to buy any. In these cases, acquiring a wardrobe depends on the home's supply and the staff's generosity: "I spent $200 out of my own pocket. She had no clothes at all" (head nurse, Court).

Obtaining, securing and spending money can be more problematic than maintaining a wardrobe. The state welfare program pays $30 a month as a personal care allowance to the resident. For most residents, this is the only source of income. There are a few exceptions, but the amount of additional money is generally small. For example, the kitchen staff chips in a little money every month for the residents who helps them: "I do a few chores and they give me a nickel or a dime. Plus I get a little money from my beano winnings (Ella, Court). Problems in obtaining the personal allowance are a common complaint among patients. Few of them actually receive $30 in cash at the first of the month. A home sometimes holds the money until it is requested by the resident, or hands it out in weekly installments.

> He's angry about everything, money, for instance. We don't give it to him anymore at the first of the month because he cashes his check, spends the money, and for the rest of the month wants to know, "Where's my dough?" (staff nurse, Bank)

> If we give her $30, she spends it all at once, then doesn't have anything left for the rest of the month. So we give her $10 at a time. When her money is spent we show her her signatures in the book, and she says it's a forgery. (staff nurse, Brady)

One resident tried for five weeks to learn the balance in her account held by the nursing home. Corporate management, not the nursing home staff, keeps the residents' money and financial records. Getting access to and satisfaction from the administrator proved impossible.

> I tried to find out from the administrator how much it cost for my clothes, but he won't tell me. He just says, "I know, I have your case." Oh, he's a smart bird. I can't get heads or tails out of my financial situation. Why doesn't he tell me? I'm not stupid, I'm not a mental case. (Katie, Court)

Some families are also accused by nursing home staff of coming on the first of every month to pick up their relatives' personal care allowance and keep it for themselves.

Nursing home corporations have a vested financial interest in holding their residents' allowances. Besides outright theft of the allowance, the large nursing home corporation can also benefit from the money in the following way:

> Take the Thompson chain, for example. They have 27 homes in the state, and say an average of 100 patients in each. Out of 2,700 beds, say they have 2,000 welfare patients. At $30 a month for each patient, they're getting $60,000 a month. With one running account invested in long-term certificates, that's a lot of interest free and clear. Plus, if at tax time they claim that money belongs to 2,000 patients, no one pays any taxes on the derived income. (supervisor, welfare)

Securing money and valuables in an institutional setting is a notorious problem:

> I was saving my money for a cake, and somebody stole it. But what can you do about it. Nothing! (Terry, Court)

I can't keep my money *here.* I wouldn't even try it. It's not safe. (Katie, Court)

Ella keeps her money in a bag hung around her neck, and Nellie keeps a sock pinned to the inside of her dress, under her arm. The residents accuse each other and the staff of stealing. The staff attributes such complaints to the accusers' forgetfulness or confusion, and does not investigate: "She says her money is missing. I just tell her, "It's OK—don't worry about it—we'll get it back. You tell them that, and it keeps them from worrying" (attendant, Court).

Spending money is also a problem. Most residents don't have enough money to spend. Thirty dollars does not go very far. Other residents who want to buy clothes, go shopping, and so on are not physically able to get to Main Street, and nearest commercial area. Some residents have "no needs," and therefore do not spend any money at all. This presents the home with a rather unexpected problem.

> Emerson's problem is that he has too much money. He's been here for seven years. He doesn't smoke, and he has no regular expenses so he's accumulated more than $1,400 in his personal allowance account. His savings now disqualify him for welfare. (head nurse, Court)

According to one welfare department supervisor, the department discourages homes from taking the resident off the welfare rolls until his account is sufficiently depleted by nursing home costs, then reapplying, because of the processing costs. So Emerson became a consumer : "We'd buy him a color television set, but he already has one. That's the best way to reduce an account. This time I took him out, and bought him an entire new wardrobe; spent over $200. Now he wants a fancy watch too" (head nurse, Court).

An awkward ethical dilemma arises. What should be done when one resident has "too much money" and another has no money but is in need of clothes, shoes, and so on? Administrators do have the means to make "adjustments":

> The money is supposedly in a trust fund for the patient, and an itemized account is kept. But the account can be generalized. If you use words like "clothes," you can cover a multitude of sins. Many patients can't write their own name, they just put an "X" or someone helps them. So the nursing home actually controls the account. (night supervisor, Court)

A welfare department supervisor offered the following hypothetical situation:

> Say you have Loretta here with no shoes and no allowance, and old Charlie over here has $1,000 in his account. So Charlie loses $30, and Loretta gets

a pair of shoes. Somehow or other she's got to get those shoes. The home is not spuriously using his money, and it is in the best interests of a client, so why not? I'm certainly not going to complain. (welfare supervisor)

Food

According to public health nurses, the poor quality of food is the most common complaint from nursing home residents. The critics claim:

> The food is awful. These places are supposed to have a dietician, but you never see them. (retired nursing home caretaker)

> We filed a complaint when they stopped serving two eggs for breakfast. The director got the order from the company: cut back on food expenses. (welfare supervisor)

The nursing home responds: "We get $1.50 a day to feed Medicaid patients. It can't be done. Fortunately we have private patients who pick up the slack in the food bill" (head nurse, Holst).

Meal time is an institutional, not a social event. There is no pretense that meals are a time to relax and converse with friends. Food trays come up on a dumb waiter. The nurse calls out names, and residents pick up their trays and return to their rooms. With the exception of two ladies who eat in the lobby, the residents eat alone beside their beds. Residents return their own trays to the dumb waiter. They segregate plates, bowls, plastic glasses, and silverware, and scrape their leftovers into the garbage. This aspect of nursing home life best exemplifies the simplified choice between institutional efficiency and social amenities.

For the staff, feeding confused patients requires special attention. They usually have unconventional eating habits and tastes.

> She eats jello with her fingers, and the sandwich with a spoon. (night supervisor, Court)

> Agnes! Stop eating with that napkin! (staff nurse 1, Court)

> Ed (resident): What's this?
> Head Nurse: It's rice.
> Ed: I don't like it dry.
> Head nurse: We'll put some gravy on it.
> Ed: What's this?
> Head nurse: Ground pork chop.
> Ed: I don't want it ground.
> Head nurse: Last week you insisted on having it ground.
> [The head nurse ordered a new tray with gravy on the rice and no ground

meat. A minute later Ed walked out the front door.] He'll wait until he knows I've ordered a new tray, then he'll go for a walk. I let him get away with it. (Court)

Accomplishing the Toilet

If there is a problem in managing routine toilet needs, the residents are labeled "incontinent." Nursing home staff usually attributes incontinence to personality or social mechanisms rather than to physiological disability:

> The incontinent patient gets a lot of extra attention because of bed wetting. The continent patients see this, and they become incontinent. I've seen one patient do this to an entire room. Sometimes it will work the other way. The single incontinent patient will get embarrassed so he'll ask for a bedpan. I just wait and see which way it will go, and then make the necessary adjustments. (head nurse, Court)

> When she has something to do, when she's stimulated, she's not incontinent. (head nurse, Holst)

If nursing home routine is disrupted for such events as an all-day outing to the amusement park, managing the toilet is a problem for every resident. At the amusement park pavilion, a portable commode was set up, and partially shielded by a screen. Although this arrangement left the resident exposed to onlookers, the commode was constantly in use: "Bringing along that portable commode is the best thing we've ever done. We've already emptied it twice this morning" (head nurse, Court). Another nursing home event, the remotivation therapy session, must be terminated early each week because four or five of the nine resident participants have urinated during the session.

For the resident who is physically restrained, there may be no management of toilet: "Fred, the wanderer, was tied to his chair, wearing only a shirt, sweater, and hat. He strained his bonds, sat up on the arm of the chair, and urinated across the floor" (observation).

SELECTION, DISCIPLINE, DISCHARGE

In addition to the routine and inevitable staff-resident conflicts, "management problem" or "behavior problem" residents are particularly troublesome to the staff. For example, occasional incontinence is a routine problem, but the resident who consistently defecates in closets is a management problem. A resident who wanders off once in a while is not the same as a chronic escapee. Although nursing homes are usually considered residential settings for physically disabled or convalescing patients, many studies show that deviant behavior is one of the most critical problems facing nursing home personnel (Stotsky 1970).

Social scientists (Goffman 1959; Stannard 1973; Curtin 1973; Rosenhan 1973) assert that the source of the staff-resident conflict is in the nature of the institution itself. Institutional efficiency causes the conflict, and necessitates the suppression of deviance and disruption. But nursing home personnel perceive themselves as humanistic caretakers of the elderly, rather than tools of institutional efficiency. Through selective admission, discipline, and discharge of the incorrigibles, they are able to minimize disruption and foster a reconciliation between practice and ideology.

Protecting the quality of life for all residents is a worthy objective and exclusionary rationale used by nursing home staff as well as professionals:

> We can't take too many of the state hospital patients. They're disruptive, and we want to make things as "homey" as possible. (head nurse, Holst)

> The nursing home must respect the interests of their residents and the pressure of their families. If my mother were in a home, I wouldn't want Mary [the screamer] in a room with her. (Social worker 1, CSH)

> Mixing the mental weakness patients with the better functioning is the primary problem in the nursing home today. (private physician 3)

The staff's explanation is reiterated by residents who do not like having to put up with their confused counterparts.

> I know she has a problem, and there's nothing to be done about it, but still you got to sleep at night. Enough is enough. (Mary, Court)

> Someone told me that if you mix with mental people you get to be like them after a while. Is that true? (Katie, Court)

The scope of the residents' problems varies from the usual noisy nights to the possibility of extreme defilement:

> [Ella was crying because her room was ransacked while she was out. The nurse calmed her.] Nothing was missing. Don't let it get you down. Don't cry. We can't watch everyone. Some people just get confused, and don't know what they're doing. (night supervisor, Court)

> Because he urinates in water pitchers, I can't have any in a room where he is. Some of the men won't tolerate that. He's lucky. One of his roommates covers the clothes in his drawer in case Ed ever decides to urinate in the drawer. (staff nurse, Bank)

Tolerance for a particular kind of problem patient varies from home to home. Some homes are thought to show a greater willingness to "work with patients" than others. The critical behaviors (Stotsky 1970) include wandering, flailing or combativeness, swearing, sexual misconduct, and incontinence.

> Some homes, if a patient yells they send them back. But the Brady, they really work with theirs. They're even keeping an assaultive patient, and I've never seen that before. (psychiatric nurse 1, CSH)

> If you swear in a Catholic-sponsored home, you're out. (psychiatric nurse 1, GST)

> One nurse is always calling with sexual misconduct complaints. She has a man who wanderers into the ladies' rooms, and she thinks he should be castrated. (community psychiatrist)

Whether or not a home accepts and keeps a candidate also depends on the nature of the relationship with the placement institution, and relationship with the patient, and extenuating circumstances such as extreme age or critical illness.

> If City Hospital continuing care tells me, I know it's a problem patient. I'll accept them because I know they'll work with me. They'll come out. They'll make the transfer if necessary. (head nurse, Court)

> The cooperative, appreciative patient becomes a pet. They'll tolerate a lot. They'll take a lot of time with him. The staff gets gratification from this. And they deserve all they can get. They respond personally to the patients. (social worker, Veterans' Hospital)

> Right now he's restless and confused, but he's 94, and his condition is guarded. He deserves to express himself once in awhile. (head nurse, Court)

Homes are able to be selective because there are many more candidates for admission than beds available. All placement organizations acknowledge the difficulty of finding an open bed; "I called 25 homes before I was able to place one patient" (social worker, Community Hospital). Nursing home administrators are not free to reject every inferior candidate and wait for the best. They do need to keep their beds filled. Particularly for the small level-three homes with few beds, quick replacement after resident discharge or death is a financial necessity. Furthermore, if homes expect to have the "good" candidates referred to them by the large placement institutions, they must occasionally accept a "bad" one: "In the beginning I got the worst ones, but when you have empty beds . . ." (head nurse, Court).

Admitting and keeping the problem patient reflect a home's tolerance for disruption in general or for specific behaviors, and implies its willingness to "work with that patient." This involves a self-adjustment on the part of home and staff, a pattern of spontaneous or planned-in-advance disciplinary measures, or both.

> When Peggy refuses to go to bed, we just let her stay up. She can get really wound up. We give her a lot of food to pacify her. (night supervisor, Court)

> After he began defecating in closets, we put locks on all the closet doors. (staff nurse, Bank)

> He urinates in the window at night, so we put a dresser in front of it. Sometimes he just moves the dresser. (staff nurse, Bank)

Disciplinary tactics are often specific to the nature of the behavioral violation of the home's regulations. For instance, the wanderer may lose his shoes or pants or be tied to a chair. There are other generally applicable tactics; threats and medication are the most frequently used. Discipline is considered to be a necessity or in the residents' best interests.

> We try to help them, try to discipline. If they don't want to obey the rules, that's just childishness. Sometimes they've gone back into their third or fourth childhood. Sometimes a little slap is necessary to get them back into this world. (staff nurse 1, Court)

The extent to which threats are made and carried out is uncertain. Physical violence is rare, at least at the Court. Most residents as well as staff want to avoid it.

> Resident: I'll hit you?
> Head nurse (Court): You hit me; I'll hit you back.
> Resident: You can't hit me! I'm a mental patient.
> Head nurse: If you're sane enough to hit me, I'm crazy enough to hit you back.

> The minute she saw the police, she got a real nasty attitude—swearing and threatening. She got in the back seat of the police cruiser, and wouldn't get out. We all tried coaxing her. Then she spit in my face. It's the only time I ever felt like striking a patient. I just yanked her out. She claimed brutality. The police wouldn't do anything to help me. They just stood there. (head nurse, Court)

Charles Stannard (1973) reports that physical abuse, though denied and regarded as wrong, is not novel. When the resident violates the institutional expectations of behavior—kicking, biting, or spitting on an aide—the prohibitions against patient abuse are temporarily suspended.

The use of tranquilizers in nursing homes, as in mental hospitals, is a complicated and controversial issue. Tranquilizers have been criticized as pharmacological straitjackets; they have also been associated with a tremendous decline in the violence, agitation, irritability, and noise of mental patients (Schwartz and Schwartz 1964). According to professionals, even though drugs do not cure, they do reduce the overt symptoms of mental disturbance, and therefore facilitate the patient's control, care, and treatment. The use of tranquilizers with the elderly in nursing homes clearly extends this idealized explanation into the domain of discipline:

> Given the inadequate staffing and unskilled workers, one must be pragmatic. While it may not be good, it may be necessary to control behavior. (geriatric psychiatrist)

> If I have one that is troublesome, I tranquilize. What else can I do? (private physician 3)

> The patients who have given us trouble are on "medical treatment." (head nurse, Holst)

Choice of drug, dosage, and administration may involve psychiatric consultants, a house doctor, and the nurse supervisor, or any one of these people. When a psychiatric nurse or social worker consults on a nursing home resident, she may "recommend" a tranquilizer and dosage. The house doctor then signs the order when he or she is in the home. Such recommendations may be routinely signed without question, or the signature may come weeks after the drug is recommended. If a house doctor prescribes a tranquilizer, it is usually at the head nurse's request, or at least is a result of her account of the patient's behavior. The head nurse herself can make the prescription decision.

> I'm called in the middle of the night because someone is climbing the wall. They say, "What can we do? There are no drugs on order." I tell them to look back two or three months for old orders. The next morning when I come in, I'll sign for them. I don't call doctors because they won't come. (head nurse, Holst)

> He's a little tiny guy. One milligram of Haldol is keeping him too drowsy. He really doesn't need it anyway. So I told the nurses to change the order to PRN. I want to get the doctor to change it when he comes in. (head nurse, Court)

Medication by negotiation is not uncommon:

> Psychiatric resident 12 (CSH): Give him Stellazine three times a day, and if that doesn't make him too confused, we'll raise it to four.

Head nurse (Court): Give him Stellazine with the chloral hydrate he's taking now?

Psychiatric resident 12: No, just Stellazine. Well, maybe you should try them together. Sometimes they work well together.

Psychiatric nurse 12 (CSH): Are you sure they can be used together?

Psychiatric resident 12: Oh, yes.

Even though the psychiatric consultant or house doctor may write an order for a tranquilizer, the nursing home staff does not always administer the medication. They have their own notions about the use of tranquilizers, and little confidence in the psychiatrist's judgment.

Each doctor has his own preferences in drugs. Doctors will try different pills. If no improvement with one, they'll try another in a few weeks. (head nurse, Court)

The mental health people believe in "maintenance." Well, for management, OK, give it to them. But I don't believe in it for everyone. The mental hospital staff says that maintenance is necessary because it takes tranquilizers too long to take effect in a crisis. But the body develops an immunity so they have to shift tranquilizers frequently. (head nurse, Court)

One nurse reported withholding medication as a form of discipline. If the resident is diabetic or has heart disease, the threat is a serious one: "We don't even withhold vitamins or tranquilizers here. But I was accused of that in another home. I didn't do it, but it was done" (night supervisor, Court).

It is clear that the head nurse is the most important participant in the decisions about the use of tranquilizers. The doctor's role is ceremonial. The resident to be tranquilized plays no part whatsoever in the decision to medicate.

Professionals inside and outside the home see discharge as the ultimate disciplinary tactic. D. B. Miller (1974) concluded from his study of discharges from two nursing homes that discharge was related more to unhappiness with the placement than to patient improvement.

The nursing home thinks that if they've got a problem with a patient, then he belongs somewhere else. (social worker 5, CH)

Of course if they get too bad we send them to the mental hospital. (staff nurse 1, Court)

We have a patient who wants to go out and stand in the snow. He stands in the hall screaming. He hogs the TV, so he can't go into a room with any other patient. What can I do? I want him out! (head nurse, Holst)

Community residents give similar reports:

He had a fight with another nursing home resident, so the staff sent him down to the mental hospital for a few weeks, then let him come back. Once they do that, it makes an example out of him, and makes the others behave. (chef, luncheonette)

The ones that are too noisy or too abusive, they go to a mental hospital and never come back. (retired nursing home caretaker)

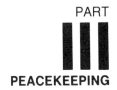

PART

III

PEACEKEEPING

Claiborne has a unique mental health team of geriatric specialists ("one of the few in the country.") The team is a part of the community mental health component at Central State Hospital, and is composed of one psychiatrist (the team leader), two full-time social workers, and one full-time and one part-time psychiatric nurse. Other pro forma or marginal participants include one volunteer, one continuing care worker from Central State Hospital, and the geriatric outreach worker. The Geriatric Specialist Team has defined its functions as consultation, training and education, and program development. It claims to perform these services in Claiborne's 30 nursing homes, elderly public housing, three neighborhood health centers, Chronic hospital, three senior citizen centers, and other community settings in need of its assistance. Claiborne is only one of several communities in its catchment area. Noticeable in its absence is any team claim to treat patients clinically: "We want to avoid seduction into taking over clinical responsibility. We've made it clear for five years that we don't do follow-up," (psychiatrist, GST).

From the team members' point of view, their operation is guided by the principles of community mental health care. The peacekeeping frame of reference encompasses their range of program action, and best typifies their performance as community agents. For example, as consultants, a role that members estimate takes 50 percent of their time,* their job is to quell disputes between

---

*I do not have accurate information as to the frequency of calls or consultations given. Team members reported that the number varies from four times a day to two times a week. In one observed conversation, psychiatric nurse 2 intimated that no calls were coming in at the present time: "Requests for consultations have stopped, period."

organizations and to quiet disruptive nursing home patients and calm their disturbed staff.

A CONCEPTUAL DILEMMA

As specialists in geriatric mental health, the team is sensitive to overuse of tranquilizers with geriatric patients and to the abuse of diagnosis when used as an excuse for rejecting and neglecting the elderly. Yet this unit's primary function is to evaluate the mental impairment of "management problems" and to recommend appropriate medication: "When we're called to nursing homes, the consultation is usually concerned with behavioral problems and medication adjustment," (psychiatric nurse 1, GST). The word "medication" is a euphemism for psychoactive drugs, and when used in conjunction with a "management problem" patient means a tranquilizer. The word "tranquilizer" is seldom used by professionals.

The unit's role and ideology are in conflict. A conceptual solution to the dilemma begins in making a distinction between "senility" and "true senility": "True senility or true organic brain syndrome, the terms can be used interchangeably. They mean the same thing; it is unremittable, irreversible. This is brain atrophy," (psychiatrist, GST). To distinguish its supposedly more accurate and, by implication, less frequent use of the term, the unit adds the adjective "true." For it, the real problem is misdiagnosis by uninformed or inexperienced professionals. When one of the specialists tranquilizes a disruptive nursing home patient, that individual is truly senile. When a nonspecialist does it, that individual is possibly falsely presumed to be senile. Ironically, the unit chooses to add the word "true" even though it does not have or regularly use medical technology necessary to directly and empirically measure brain atrophy. As will be discussed in Chapters 8 and 9, even technological assessment of brain atrophy is problematic as a scientific procedure.

The unit's assumption of greater accuracy in diagnosis is suspect since the criteria for so-called true senility are identical to those for senility: " . . . calculations are the first to go. . . . recent memory and memory in general. . . . fund of knowledge. . . . symbolic processes," (psychiatrist, GST). This is indistinguishable from the mental status exam. The false distinction sufficiently obscures the concept so that the specialists can reconcile contributing to the social abuses against which they are expected to protest. The Geriatric Specialist Team's claim to special knowledge and the definition of its own proper role combine to involve it, more than other professionals, in the diagnosis of senility and organic brain syndrome:

[GST social worker 1 made the following diagnosis of a "management problem" after a consultation in a nursing home with a psychiatric resident.]

1. Organic dementia
2. Psychosis with unknown etiology (possibly functional or organic)
3. Possible schizophrenic depression
[The treatments prescribed were Mellaril (a tranquilizer) and putting plants in his window because he was a professional gardener before retiring.]

It is the unit's job to recognize senility and to help in handling it. Also, because it steadfastly disavows all direct treatment roles and refuses to do dirty work in the community, it doesn't witness survival strategies as mitigating factors in its diagnosis. Its dilemma reemerges at each point of community intervention.

SERVICING THE MANAGERS

There are elements of choice and default in the geriatric specialists' obligation to encourage and protect peaceful working relationships among Central State Hospital, nursing homes, and other community settings. Central State Hospital expects the geriatric specialists to serve in the community as its appendage. The relationship between the hospital and the Geriatric Specialist Team, however, is not well defined and is sometimes antagonistic. As hospital employees, the geriatric specialists are cautious and hesitant to contradict or criticize their employer openly. But a basic hostility in their relationship is indicated by such generalized complaints as:

It's a very hard institution to work with. (psychiatrist, GST)

It's incest! They've all been on each other's couch. They've all been supervised and psychoanalyzed by one another. (psychiatric nurse 1, GST)

The team thinks the hospital places low priority on the needs of the elderly, and is reluctant to become involved: "There were 105 requests for staff in the new budget, and only one for a geriatric staff person. When we submitted our proposal, it was put at the bottom of the list, the last priority" (psychiatric nurse 1, GST). In return, the hospital ward staff complains about the basic function of the unit:

When they go into nursing homes they only deal with staff, not the patients. They don't want to work with patients so they don't. I think they're on some federal grant so they do just what they want to. (social worker 1, CSH)

They don't do anything to make patients better. (social worker 4, CSH)

The hospital's admission staff, however, does not have any complaints.

They can call on the unit to act as intermediary between a nursing home and the hospital when a home wants to admit a resident:

The geriatric specialists' contribution is in reducing admissions. (psychiatric resident 11, CSH)

When we get a call from a home, we ask them to hold the patient until we can get a geriatric specialist there. We depend on them for early intervention to avoid hospitalization. (psychiatric resident 2, CSH)

Stated in idealized terms, the fundamental peacekeeping role of the unit is

They can prevent the mutual mistrust between home and hospital from getting too far out of hand. Nursing homes need to know that they can appeal here and get a response. And we must be able to believe a nursing home when they say they will take back a patient after he is restabilized. (psychiatric resident 2, CSH)

The team acknowledges the popular conception of nursing homes as bureaucratic institutions that depersonalize the resident with inferior, custodial handling. It is generally critical of nursing homes as residences for confused elderly:

Nursing homes are no place for senile dementia patients. The staff isn't trained. They infantilize patients. We need to change their attitude. (psychiatric nurse 1, GST)

The staff doesn't know anything about mental health, and they're afraid of mental health workers. (psychiatric nurse 1, GST)

As practitioners, they are obliged to serve the individual, and in the abstract, they tend to sympathize with the residents:

Swearing is another behavior that homes won't tolerate. But I think patients should swear back, and some of them do. (psychiatric nurse 1, GST)

Generally they want to quiet a noisy patient. He may be noisy because he's the character with a little life left in him. When I tell the nurses this, it's not what they want to hear. They want to sedate him. (psychiatric nurse 2, GST)

Yet, establishing and maintaining a working relationship with some 30 nursing homes in Claiborne (as well as the rest of the catchment area) occupies the largest part of the geriatric specialists' time.
Nursing homes call on the team for advice in handling management problems.

The team's primary association is with the home management, not the resident. Serving the confused elderly is confused with serving the management. If GST practitioners confront the nursing home and challenge the home's definition of the problem by siding with the patient, they risk losing the home as a consultee. The following complaint illustrates the resentment of the nursing home when the mental health specialist refused to accept the home's explanation of the situation or to comply with their expectations.*

> We called after we found the lady hanging over the railing. We regard that as an attempted suicide, which is a committable offense. And we wanted her committed. They refused to commit her, and said there was no suicide attempt. And after listening to her complaints about the evening staff, they criticized us. *How could they possibly know the real situation after talking with her for only a few minutes?* They were no help at all. (private physician, Charity Nursing Home)

The superficiality of the consultation mechanism is criticized only when the home is dissatisfied. Resident dissatisfaction is not even an issue because they are excluded from the decision making and given no opportunity to complain.

Since the geriatric specialists want to protect their relationship with the nursing home, they must rely on the staff's veracity and discount the presumed senile individual's report as confused and unreliable. Not only do the specialists refuse to consider the validity of a specific complaint by residents, such as the common accusation of stealing, but they provide a rationale for ignoring it: "When they realize they can't remember what they did with something, then it's easier for them to complain about it being stolen than to blame their own memory," (psychiatric nurse 1, GST). Charges against the staff are described as "distortion" or as an "isolated event when someone lost his temper." In the absence of empirical evidence, such explanations constitute loyalty statements. The discrepancies between their general allegiance to the individual and their responses to specific situations are rationalized by their perception of rendering service to the staff, which, in turn, benefits the residents.

> They're genuinely appreciative. They're worried about patients and their families complaining and moving out, and the resultant lost revenue. (psychiatrist, GST)

---

*I did not observe or hear of occasions when the geriatric specialists challenged the nursing home's account. This incident is not a reference to the GST but to the consultant from another Community Mental Health Center. Interestingly, this confrontation came when commitment was the issue rather than medication, and when the consultant's own interests were at stake.

We try to make the situation more tenable for the nurse in order to make it better for the patient. (psychiatric nurse 1, GST)

In the "good" nursing homes (those that participate in the training program) where team members have established rapport, their allegiance to home staff has credibility, at least to them. In homes considered inferior, they resort to deliberate inattention rather than intervene. A nursing home had been accused of negligence by the team, and blacklisted by Public Hospital when one of three recently placed hospital patients had died after rapid deterioration. The team pondered its obligation to expose the home.

Psychiatric nurse 1: Our expertise isn't physical. We can't take responsibility for that.
Psychiatrist: But we are doctors and nurses.
Psychiatric nurse 1: Find someone else; it ain't me.
Social worker 1: If we squeal, will we be able to use the home again, or do we want to?
Psychiatric nurse 1: They aren't confronted because no one wants to put them on the defensive.
Social worker 1: So what if they get angry or upset?
Psychiatric nurse 1: They still have two of our patients there. We don't know that they would take revenge on them, but we must protect them.

As mental health practitioners, the GST supposedly serves patients, but for the programmatic reasons just discussed, it services nursing home staff who handles the patients. The direction of the service is not in question. When the geriatric specialists are approached, however, by an unfamiliar community organization, the choice of "client" is ambiguous and subject to debate. A tenants' council, for example, wanted to keep as many people as possible in a building after a mass eviction notice by the owners. The council requested GST's help with a confused elderly lady in the building who had become a nuisance with her constant telephone calls. The GST staff observed a conflict between its "clinical" role and "community organization" role: "If she chooses to leave, you can't be for the cause and the lady both," (psychiatrist, GST). The issue was complicated because team members wanted to take into consideration the cause, the extent of the lady's distress, and the intentions of the council.

The council's cause is a worthy one. They are trying to prevent the dislocation of many low income and elderly people. Does it justify the lady's distress?
They must judge the extent of the lady's fear, and interpret her conflicting and ambiguous statements.

Does the council really want help or just publicity in their struggle against the owner? Does it "smack of secret police"?

From the point of view of the local stations in the community, particularly those doing community dirty work, the geriatric specialists don't have much to offer:

> We work with patients and people who deal with patients. The geriatric specialists are concerned with policy, the bigger issues. We get along without them, and this is all right. (geriatric workshop leader)

> They're just trying to keep patients out of the hospital. (nurse, Visiting Nurse Association)

Consultation, training and education, and program development are redefinitions of the classical clinical role, but consistent with the Community Mental Health Center's ideology. Such redefinitions constitute a reality adjustment of the mental health practitioner. The geriatric specialists' assigned tasks illustrate the point. These professionals were trained as clinicians in psychiatry, nursing, and social work, but refuse to do clinical treatment. On one hand, they face the problem of being specialists in the treatment of people they themselves define as being beyond rehabilitation, the unremittably, irreversibly confused older person. They choose to replace clinical treatment with peacekeeping and policing skills. Their primary social role as peacekeepers is better accommodated by the consultation-education-training frame of reference than by the model of clinical practice. Working relationships are established with social agents, not patients. Therefore a consultative model is necessary to define their new reciprocal role relationships. While a senior citizen center director may resist being identified as the trainee, the role of "patient" would be totally unacceptable. The reality adjustment gives the team an ideology that approximates its function and is generally acceptable to its associates.

STRATEGIES FOR POLICING INDIVIDUALS

Through their professional contacts, geriatric specialists extend their peacekeeping actions to surveillance of confused elderly on the street. Community agents (for example, senior citizen center directors) regularly report on the behavior and condition of certain potentially troublesome seniors. Psychiatric nurses from the Geriatric Specialist Team attend the senior citizen center lunches once a week; this is frequent enough to keep up to date on behavior problems, but not often enough to get to know the seniors themselves. In the absence of routine personal involvement with center members, team function evolves into surveillance and the application of moral sanctions against deviants. The surveillance nature of their work is best characterized by the observation of one senior member:

> They come for a chitchat, then go. . . . Now she's a wonderful girl but she'd come once and you wouldn't see her again for a couple of weeks. They don't put in enough time to follow through. You can't get too much of a grasp on things with the time they spend around here. For a long time I thought they were collecting information for some headquarters. (senior citizen 7)

As previously described, the seniors tend to be intolerant of the nonconforming or "graceless" members. The geriatric specialists lend the weight of professional authority to the seniors' discriminatory interests, and therefore legitimize exclusionary practices. "The senior citizens are furious. And they should be. She's resigned herself to pighood for life, and she should be removed from the center," (psychiatric nurse 2, GST). The specialists themselves are middle class, like the seniors they visit, and share the social conventions of the center's participants. By virtue of their professional credentials, they become a source of explanation and rationale for mutually held standards of behavior, and an authority that enforces conformity: "The very confused don't want to go to the centers. They recognize their inadequacy, and withdraw, refusing to participate. They don't come because they know they can't handle it," (psychiatric nurse 1, GST).

Nursing home consultation is intended to be a crisis intervention operation. Nursing homes are encouraged to call when there is an emergency. The operation is usually carried out in two stages. A geriatric specialist, either a nurse or social worker (not the psychiatrist), responds to the nursing home's call about a management problem. She surveys the situation and makes plans to return with a psychiatric resident if the patient does not improve. The outcome of either visit, but usually the second, is tranquilization.

> We're called for consultation when the patient's behavior makes the staff anxious, that is, the management problems. (social worker, GST)

> When we're called to a nursing home, the consultation is usually concerned with behavioral problems and medication adjustment. (psychiatric nurse 1, GST)

The first stage is devoted to a reconstruction of reality. For reasons already elaborated in the discussion of the nursing home specialist association, this reconstruction converts the staff's complaints into psychiatric jargon that locates the origin of the problem in the resident's mental state.

> [For six months, Marilyn, a resident, has been ill at ease in the home. She complains about her peers, and is afraid of being discharged. The night

before she went out and got drunk. A geriatric specialist was called for a consultation. Her observation]: She has a little brain damage. She's been acting up lately but we really don't know why. She's confused. (social worker, GST)

The second stage is demarcated by a medication adjustment. The specialist herself or a psychiatric resident from Central State Hospital recommends the drug and its dosage. It is important for the nurse or social worker specialist to have a psychiatric resident participate in this phase. Residents, however, are reluctant. They consider nursing home consultation to be outside their proper domain, and they lack any hospital supervision. Furthermore, they have no continuing relationship or responsibility to the nursing home or patient.

[To geriatric specialist]: I can tell you in advance that I can't do anything. I haven't any experience with this kind of thing. I think you might want a neurology consult. (psychiatric resident 1, CSH)

Residents don't want to go to nursing homes because there's no backup. They are the senior person on the case. (psychiatric resident 2, CSH)

The psychiatric residents are also vulnerable to physical and social defilements that would be unlikely to occur in the hospital.

Just before I arrived he had a copious bowel movement in bed. When I entered the room, he began throwing his feces at me. I stood there, naked to the waist, consulting with the staff while my shirt was being laundered. (psychiatric resident 2, CSH)

In another case, the psychiatric resident interviewed a patient who was afraid of the staff. She whispered about threats made against her and about her confiscated money. He steadfastly refused to take up her complaints, and instead insisted that she come to the hospital for an appointment. During this conversation, a threat to the patient in the next room was overheard:

Male voice: Were you in the kitchen?
Female elderly voice [hesitantly]: Yes.
Male voice: You go in there again when I'm cleaning, I'm gonna choke you.

The psychiatric resident later admitted that he had heard the threat, but decided not to respond to it. Because the nature of the resident's function is not treatment, but peacekeeping, he was forced to act out a social delusion: that he didn't hear a threat to a patient, that his patient's complaints were not corroborated, and that he was not obligated to confront the home with the complaints or the evidence. Instead, he made this analysis:

This type of mildly paranoid delusional personality [at the hospital she thought the intercom speaker was a microphone recording her voice] doesn't respond well to authority, even when it's only the slightest bit of repression, the sort that is universally present in any sort of institutional environment. (psychiatric resident 4, CSH)

Tranquilization is invariably the outcome of the consultation and, in a sense, its ultimate purpose. It is prescribed without any planned follow up or any other simultaneous treatment. While the specialists recommend that someone on the staff "get involved with the patient," they do not offer (and therefore tacitly refuse) to take the responsibility themselves. Success is equated with the absence of future complaint. Under these circumstances, the consultation is clearly a peacekeeping operation.

The GST holds seminars once a month for nursing home staff. The same two specialists run each seminar in Claiborne. Seminars are conducted in rotation at the participating nursing homes. One home is assigned to present "a case." The following is a summary of a management problem case presented at a seminar:

He can't find the bathroom. He can't find his own bed. He collects water pitchers. He has an obsession about food. He complains if the meal is a minute late, and watches the clock constantly. He urinates on the floor and in the windowsill, and defecates in the linen closet. But he's not incontinent. If you tell him he's doing something wrong, he gets angry. We don't let him cash his check anymore because he spends all his money, and accuses us of keeping it. He's abusive. He denounces all the black nurses and attendants.

The seminar is significant as a social event with performances and audiences, but not as a mechanism for diagnosis and treatment of a specific management problem. In fact, the forum exposes the consultant's confusion. For example, the specialist's conclusion to the above case was:

He's angry. He's furious. Did anything happen two or three months ago? Maybe he's depressed. Depression causes memory loss. Maybe he needs antidepression medication. [He is receiving antidepression medication.] His diagnosis is chronic brain syndrome, and he's an old alcoholic. He has Korsakoff's syndrome, and it's progressive. That's treated with vitamins. Maybe he needs vitamins. He may be getting hardening of the arteries. He should have a physical. He may be like Frank, and there just isn't much you can do. He likes to eat; maybe he can help with the food. (psychiatric nurse 1, GST)

The chief accomplishment of the seminar is the exchange of social supports. The presenting home has the opportunity to elaborate what a good job it had done, and it is the social responsibility of the others to congratulate and encourage. Peacekeeping is indirectly accomplished by buoying the spirits of the oppressed nursing home staff.

> Presentation: We moved him to a new room, closer to the bathroom. We tried waking him up every two hours in the night to use the toilet, but he became too agitated. We put a dresser in front of the window and locks on all the cabinets. There are signs pointing to the toilet. He's on Hydergene, and we're paying for it—$2.70 a day worth of free medication. (staff nurse, Bank Nursing Home)
>   Response: How have you been able to put up with this? We'd never be able to. (staff nurse, Holst Nursing Home)
>   It's remarkable that you've been so tolerant. How much longer can you go on? (staff nurse, Clover Nursing Home)

The staff's manufacturing of this supportive process out of the event is intrinsic evidence of its value to them. (Since seminar participation is dwindling, it may be that another format would better serve the same purpose.)

The inevitable consequence of the seminar as well as the consultation is a "medication adjustment," and these strategies take on the appearance of ritualistic exercises that stage the prescription of tranquilizing drugs. The appearance of the psychiatric resident also has ceremonial qualities. Medications can be ordered without him, and he has no further responsibility to the patient. The nursing home resident does not become *his* patient. The problem is expressed by one team specialist: "We take out residents who write prescriptions for phenothiozenes without termination. So the patient stays on them for life," (psychiatric nurse 2, GST).

One incidental achievement of the consultation and seminar is that nursing home staff is trained in the use of the myth of futility. It is the specialists and psychiatric residents who introduce ideas about irreversible impairment to nonprofessionals as a way of handling their problems.

> Psychiatric nurse 2 [after a nursing home consultation]: I thought there would be something we could do. It's just a fantasy.
>   Psychiatric resident 1: We did do something. We helped the nursing home staff to see that nothing could be done.*

---

*Ironically, the following report was given to me on this nursing home resident seven weeks after this consultation: "He's doing just fine now. He's in a room with a blind man, and *he* takes the blind man to the bathroom, and waits for him to come out" (staff nurse, Bank Nursing Home).

CHAPTER

7

THE POLICEMEN

The point of view of the police emphasizes the harmless and fragile nature of the confused elderly. They may be a nuisance on the street, an occasional inconvenience to the policeman in the routine performance of his duties, but they are not criminals. The police most frequently come into contact with confused elderly through street surveillance. A typical encounter involves transporting a lost or wandering old person to the nursing home, City Hospital, Central State Hospital, or occasionally to private residences. The policeman's peacekeeping contribution is best understood by examining first the policeman's view of his job and then the pattern of recurring encounters with the confused elderly, with the nursing homes, and with Central State Hospital.

The Claiborne police describe themselves as a public service organization: "Eighty percent of the work we do is aid and assist. Maybe 10 percent of our work is criminal" (captain). The police know their community. They are familiar with the location of all the nursing homes. They know the confused elderly street regulars on sight. They eat breakfast and lunch at the luncheonette where confused elderly hang out, and they know the common street names applied to some of the eccentrics. In fact, one motorcycle patrolman "deputized" an elderly man who pretended to be a policeman, and gave him an old police shirt. He was known as "the Deputy." "They can be spotted. We know them all. We notice right away if there's a new one" (captain). This familiarity is useful to the police in their job of protecting Main Street's commercial stability and tranquility. They know the "smokers" who are always bumming cigarettes. The police perform a "public service" in keeping them off Main Street.

Police are reluctant to pursue even the more serious offenders with formal police action. It would be inconsistent with their role as friendly public servants to arrest old people for their offenses.

One old man gave me the finger so I stopped him. He said, "I was just saying hi." I let him go. (policeman 2)

We had one old man just released from the state hospital. He'd been in for 18 or 20 years. He was whoopin' and hollerin' on the streets, and ringing doorbells. We had three or four calls. But what could we do? You can't charge someone with ringing doorbells. (captain)

POLICE AND CONFUSED ELDERLY

Maintaining good community relations is, by definition, a part of the police's job, and they are particularly sensitive to complaints from the community. The interests of community members with the social power of complaint, such as nursing home and hospital staff and landlords, must be taken into account. Since confused elderly have little power of complaint, their preferences and point of view are not taken seriously, however genially police may regard them.

The services confused elderly request interfere with the policeman's duty. For example, police are prepared for the emergency and the crisis. They want to be ready to answer a first aid call at any time. From their point of view, taxiing the elderly, particularly lost or wandering nursing home residents, is inconsistent with their role and potentially obstructive to their state of readiness.

The problem is when you get an emergency call and you have an elderly person in the car. You can't take him along. What can you do? You have to give him immediate shelter. If it's winter, you put him in a store and have the management watch him. Then you come back later and pick him up. (policeman 2)

When the police cannot avoid direct involvement, they minimize the time and content of the exchange. In the following illustration, a confused elderly lady with no where to go attempted to escape from a nursing home. Apparently hoping to dodge a home attendant in pursuit, she entered the police station.

Police Sergeant [in a gruff, inhospitable tone]: What's she doing here (to the attendant)? Does she belong to you? Why did you let her out?
Lady: I belong to myself!
Attendant: She's from the Autumn Nursing Home.
Police Sergeant: Ralph! Get a car, and drive her to 20 Pearl Street.

This attendant analyzed the sergeant's attitude: "Basically he's a nice man. But you know, she's an old lady, and he just didn't want to be bothered. He has other things to do" (attendant, Autumn). In front of the nursing home, the lady refused to get out of the police cruiser, and, when finally coaxed out, she refused to enter the home. The attendant and one policeman gently but firmly pushed her into the home. The lady insisted that the police stay, but one of them responded: "We just got a radio call that we have to answer. Don't worry, you go in, and we'll be back in ten minutes" (policeman 4). The police never returned.

This lady had no credibility with the police. Her mere appearance at police headquarters was evidence that she ought to be returned to the home. They made no inquiries about her reasons for leaving or for refusing to return. The sergeant treated her brusquely and the patrolman lied to her. Public service functioned in the interests of the home and at the expense of the lady's preferences.

Police see themselves as too busy with more important matters to make such encounters "unnecessarily" complicated. By minimizing the time lost, they can more quickly return to their real job. From their point of view, their only responsibility as defined by police procedure is limited to providing transportation: "All we do is transport them. It's no problem for police procedure" (captain).

POLICE AND THE NURSING HOME

The two major issues that bring the police and the nursing home together are the protection of nursing home property and the return of wandering residents. The police claim to do their job well, and are proud of their good relations with the nursing homes: "We get along good with the nursing homes. Excellent relations, excellent!" (captain). It is not their job to police nursing homes for violations of regulations, so their relationship is not adversarial. The police are not opposed to doing occasional peacekeeping favors for home management:

> One time I answered a call from a home. There were two ex-mental hospital patients fighting. I told them, "Either get out or I'm going to lock you up." That was just what the owner wanted to hear. It worked too—they left. He said they could come back in a few days when they realized what a good deal they had. (policeman 2)

One informant suggested another factor that influences police attitudes and performance:

> One Christmas I saw 10 or 12 cops come in asking for the administrator. They were all getting their "fifth." In return, if anything goes wrong, the

cops get there right away. Good protection is important because this is a bad neighborhood. (retired nursing home caretaker)

Nursing home personnel, however, are critical of police performance. They feel vulnerable because they have large quantities of drugs and some money. Claiborne's inner-city location and the specter of high crime rates in bad neighborhoods cause concern among the staff who feel police do not give adequate protection.

One night I called the police because I heard noises in the basement. They never came. I called back an hour later. When they finally came, they found someone had tried to pry open the basement door. But the cops were pretty well loaded by that time of the morning. All they did was raid the refrigerator. At least the thieves didn't take anything. The police took sandwiches. (head nurse, Court)

Some police are employed in their off-duty hours by nursing homes.

My job was to figure out which aides were stealing supplies, which weren't doing any work, and to keep the place quiet. Kids would come in off the street to buy soda in the vending machine. They made a racket. Almost all the homes have some kind of night watchman. (policeman 2)

These police give favorable evaluations of the nursing homes:

I've never seen any physical violence whatsoever in three years. Maybe yelling once in a while, but that's it. (policeman 2)

The homes feed the patients well. They all look clean and healthy. (policeman 5)

The night staff does not reciprocate the praise of the moonlighting policemen: "They're no good to you. How can anybody work 20 hours a day? They've got to sleep sometime, so they do it at night in the home. And when you need them, they're never there" (head nurse, Court).

When nursing homes lose residents because they run away or get lost, they expect the police to search for, find, and return them. The staff is convinced that a wandering resident is in danger, and anything other than prompt police response is neglect of duty. The police, on the other hand, are not convinced of the imminent danger to the wanderer's or escapee's life. They suspect he is having a good time and will eventually return of his own accord.

They get bored and tired of being confined. So they go out for a little scenery and beer. (policeman 3)

They're nobody's fool. They go for a five-mile walk, and want a ride back to the home. They may not look like they know what they're doing, but they always get back in time for dinner. (captain)

Given this point of view, the police do not take the swift, decisive action the homes want. Their approach is more casual.

We investigate a call before we turn it in to headquarters as a missing person. (policeman 1)

If there's a car here, we send it out to look for the wanderer. It's all procedural. If we find them, we take them back. But they usually come back on their own. (captain)

Needless to say, the nursing home considers this an unsatisfactory response:

The police make me so mad. I called them when Mrs. Liter wandered off. She'd been gone an hour, and they said, "Call back later if she's still missing." That doesn't make any sense. The longer you wait, the further they get. (head nurse, Court)

When I called to report her missing, the police said she isn't legally missing until she's been gone 24 hours. They wouldn't do anything. (staff nurse 1, Court)

THE POLICE AND CENTRAL STATE HOSPITAL

As peacekeepers, the police are called upon to answer landlord and neighborhood complaints against confused elderly. These elderly are accused of such things as wandering in the streets at night, picking through trash, ringing doorbells, and disturbing other tenants with noise and obnoxious odors from their apartments. When the landlords or neighbors are sufficiently distressed, they demand that the confused individual be removed. In some cases, the police surgeon or a community physician (or the house doctor in the nursing home) signs a commitment order. The police are expected to transport the deviant to Central State Hospital.

We answered the neighbor's complaint, and found this old lady alone in her house. She had snow tires in the kitchen, rats, mattresses all over the place. The house was a mess. You just couldn't believe it. We called the police surgeon, and he recommended taking her to Central State. (policeman 1)

Even under those circumstances, the police were hesitant to become involved in transporting. They believe that Central State Hospital consistently refuses to admit old people: "Usually Central State won't admit them. It takes two doctors to get someone committed, even if you have commitment papers signed. You have to have two signatures, one outside and one hospital doctor" (policeman 1).

The police complain of unnecessary delays and of the doctors' disregard for the policeman's observations of the home situation:

> Sometimes you have to wait two hours at Central State while they decide what to do. It doesn't pay to complain. You don't want to be responsible for bad relations. I might say, "We can't tie up a wagon this long," but that's it. (policeman 1)

> We see the patient at home. We know what he's like. The police officer's report should be given more weight. We tell the doctors he's jeopardizing other tenants' safety, and they say to us, "Are you the doctor? Can you diagnose this person?" (policeman 3)

Not only must the police deal with what they consider to be an uncooperative institution, but their failure to get satisfaction damages their prestige in the community and exposes the landlord and tenants to unnecessary risks. When the hospital refuses to admit the evicted elderly person, he must be returned to his place of residence.

> Central State refused to take her. The landlord almost died when we brought her back. He said, "You mean you can't do anything at all?" I told him, "No. There's no crime. We can't lock her up. It used to be we had more authority, but not any more." You know, we look bad in his eyes. It's no good for our relations with the community. (policeman 3)

> Central State said she's not dangerous to herself. So now we wait for something to happen. Wait until she kills herself or somebody else by burning down the building. Then it will be too late. (policeman 1)

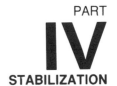

PART

IV

STABILIZATION

CHAPTER

8

THE MENTAL
HOSPITAL

Although Central State Hospital recently became a community mental health center, its psychodynamic orientation and its institutional identity as a teaching hospital have not been altered perceptibly.* Both hospital staff and outsiders agree that community mental health is only a minor component in the hospital program:

> This hospital has always been oriented towards psychodynamics of psychiatry. The old guard are not in the forefront of community psychiatry. (psychiatric resident 2, CSH)

> This is a community mental health center on paper only. It's a stepchild of the hospital. The old director never pretended to relate to the community. You can at least give him credit for that. (community health worker, PH)

Community agents complain about undeveloped hospital-community association, including admission and placement practices (to be discussed in the following pages). Even hospital employees stationed in the community say they have no formal means of entering their case records into the inpatient service:

---

*Although traditional and intransigent, the hospital was apparently in a state of transition. The director retired, and the new head had not yet been appointed. There was staff speculation about who it would be, and what changes he would make. The secret disdain for community work may have limited generalizability. The conflict between impressions and preferences is at least worth looking into in other converted state mental hospitals.

You go to the admission secretary, and put your notes on her desk. Your paper will go on one of her piles. She might remember, and she might not. They have a strictly hospital point of view. A patient isn't a patient until he walks into the hospital. (psychiatrist, GST)

Psychiatric nurse 1 (GST) accused the walk-in clinic staff of holding patients illegitimately for "extended diagnoses" because there are not enough patients to keep the staff occupied. Yet the social worker supervisor continues to refuse to give up any of these "slots" to community work: "All our community work is done behind the supervisor's back" (continuing care worker 1, CHS).

In spite of economic incentives through funding by the state department of mental health, the hospital resists adjustments toward the community.

The hospital is in bad shape. It's really shabby. What we need is a new director with political shrewdness who can get more money. Major philosophical changes will be necessary in order to get more money. (executive administrator, CSH)

They just aren't getting money for training anymore. (community health worker, PH)

The hospital's adherence to an economically maladaptive philosophy can be attributed to its teaching staff, the psychiatric residents, and the nature of psychiatric practice. The old guard determines the politics of the institution and the substance of the teaching. The institution is committed to defending its academic status in professional psychiatry.

The director wanted a basic research and training hospital. The people over there are worried that the quality of research will decline. We say if the quality is going down, it's a needed change in emphasis. But they had a national reputation, and wanted to protect it. (community health worker, PH)

The psychiatric resident's role as trainee also contributes to the anticommunity orientation.

Residents want to train for what they'll do when they get out. They don't embrace community practice because who will pay for it? Why train for what no one will pay for? (psychiatric resident 2, CSH)

I tell residents, "Go out in the community," and they answer, "All the interesting cases are in the hospital." (community health worker, PH)

Residents who want to do community work don't even apply to this hospital. (continuing care worker 2, CSH)

It has been argued in the literature that the community care movement began without theoretical rationale or logical imperatives derived from psychiatric practice (Susser 1968). Even the significance of the social environment is debated (Bauxbaum 1973). Lack of professional interest was illustrated in two reviews of professional articles on psychotherapy (Cartwright 1968; Ford and Urban 1967). Stanley Murrell (1971) pointed out that only 9 of the 244 articles reviewed were even indirectly concerned with the patients' social system. One specialist in geriatric psychiatry faults the profession's overreliance on intrapsychic dynamics and neglect of medical and social facts (Patterson 1971).* In a classic article, Kingsley Davis (1938) concluded that community or environment is neglected by psychiatry because human personality supposedly is understandable without reference to social reality. Social reality is accepted as something artificial to which the personality must adjust.

More than any other institutional attribute, Central State Hospital's role as a teaching facility defines its encounter with confused elderly and the community. The head of the hospital holds the chair in psychiatry at the affiliated university. The psychiatric residents are students and the teaching staff are faculty members at the same university. The staff psychiatrists primarily administrate, supervise residents, and hold teaching conferences.

Supervision, the core feature of training, encourages discrimination against geriatric patients because they do not fit into the prevailing treatment model.

The supervisors here are psychoanalytically oriented. They're interested in ego development, that sort of thing. And the social worker supervisor is also into dynamics. (continuing care worker 1, CSH)

Dynamic insight therapy is what the old guard want to supervise. The bulk of our elderly patients don't fall into that category. That's not a treatment for old people, per se. Residents report to supervisors the kinds of cases they want to supervise. (psychiatric resident, CSH)

Every June a new class of trainees enters and the senior class graduates. Hospital services are restaffed annually, and this rotation has a profound effect on the daily life of the institution. Continual readjustment to the arrival of new staff and the departure of old staff produce chronic instability in the hospital's

---

*Of course mental disorders have been subjects of study by many disciplines, including psychiatry, psychology, social work, psychopharmocology, anthropology, and sociology. Social deviance theory advances the opposing point of view, that mental illness is not in the quality of a normative violation in itself (the symptom) but a consequence of the environment's successful application of that label on the individual. For further reading, see Simon 1973; Thomas Scheff 1966, 1964; Becker 1963; Erikson 1962; Lemert 1972, 1951; Kitsuse 1962.

functioning. Technically, a patient is assigned to one resident at the time of admission, and this relationship is maintained until treatment is terminated, the patient withdraws, or the resident's tenure at the hospital expires. In actuality, patients do not follow their psychiatric residents from one hospital service to another. Before the residents rotate, their patients are usually terminated. A few are put on a reassignment list.

> I got a letter today from the administration saying only a few patients would be accepted for reassignment and that I would be expected to terminate with the rest. Now I'm having a hard enough time getting my active patients on the list! And what do you do with the patients no one else will take? What do you tell them when you leave and everyone else refuses to work with them? (psychiatric resident 5, CSH)

As a result, the less desirable patients who do remain on the ward no longer have an effective relationship with a psychiatric resident. The implications are obvious for the chronic geriatric patient. The academic calendar dictates the treatment agenda and experiences of a patient.

The admission process presents the same discontinuity. The residents who admit patients do not treat them and may have nothing more to do with them. This discontinuity perpetuated by the hospital's trainee assignment policy may result in arbitrary manipulation of applicants, as in the following example:

> Psychiatric resident 6: I convinced her to come for evaluation, and she was committed.
> Interviewer: Why was she committed rather than admitted?
> Psychiatric resident 6: I don't know. I left the case after she came to the hospital.

Like all social relationships, the hospital (doctor)-patient relationship is symbiotic. The patient has obvious educational utility to the institution. Exploitation is always a potential in socially symbiotic encounters, particularly when one member has greater authority and status than the other. In the hospital setting, where the doctor-patient distinction is extreme, it is said that professional standards protect the patient, but, in any event, who benefits the most is an arbitrary judgment. Discontinuity of interest as illustrated above is an unresolved problem.

ADMISSION

Statewide changes in the organization of mental health care have altered Central State Hospital's admission policy and process. Originally, the hospital selectively admitted what it considered to be the choice patients. As a community mental health center, it is now responsible for treating any resident from its catchment area. This has introduced the hospital to a new clientele. Claiborne confused elderly are directly affected.

> Only since this hospital accepted responsibility for a catchment area in conjunction with the community mental health act, has there been a push to put old people in this mental hospital. (psychiatric resident 1, CSH)

> In the past, Central State could select patients out. That meant the worst were sent to another state hospital, but it's no longer our backup. The staff doesn't want to deal with chronicity. (social worker 1, CSH)

The hospital personnel are at best skeptical about their new responsibility for handling confused elderly. They view these elderly as suffering from irreversible organic impairment, a pathology outside the domain of mental health treatment. The elderly who appear at the hospital are therefore considered misplaced:

> Old people with chronic brain syndrome are just out of it. They don't need to be in a mental hospital. It probably wouldn't do them any good. (psychiatric nurse 6, CSH)

> What could we do for that kind of person? How could you give her psychotherapy? All the psychotherapy in the world wouldn't help her. (psychiatric nurse 5, CSH)

TABLE 7
Diagnostic Categories Applicable to Confused Elderly

Functional Etiology	Organic Etiology
Involuted psychosis	Organic brain syndrome (acute and chronic)
Chronic schizophrenia	Presenile dementia (Alzheimer's disease, Pick's disease)
Depression	Senile dementia
	Senility

Screening and Diagnosis

Screening candidates is one way to evaluate an "appropriate" admission. It is also a mechanism for selecting out the undesirable (Kirk and Greenley 1974 Wiseman 1970). Because nursing home placement is difficult, and because Central State Hospital does not have a well-developed placement and follow-up operation, selective admission is essential in delimiting the patient population. The complaints of outsiders give evidence that such discrimination against undesirables, like the elderly, is practiced:

> They never want to accept anyone, anytime. Their trick is to refuse to take telephone calls from us, or refuse to release our ambulance drivers, or they refuse any referral that's not legally committable, the homicidal or suicidal. Obviously they don't refuse admission to everyone except the committable. It's a legal technicality. Not all patients in need of supervision fall into one of those categories. (psychiatrist 1, CH)

Technically, a mental health professional might identify the source of confusion in old people as functional, meaning psychological and not organic. (see Table 7) Differentiating one from the other, however, is not the purpose of diagnosis as it is practiced in the field. Diagnosis in the field addresses only the question, is the old person senile or not. On this basis, the professional will define the elderly's condition as treatable or irreversible. The presence of irreversible impairment is cause for exclusion from the hospital. In the following pages, the criteria and sources of ambiguity in diagnosis are examined.

There is no consensus among mental health professionals as to the exact definition of the organic diseases. Practitioner folk wisdom associates senility with diminished cerebral blood flow or cerebral arteriosclerosis. Organic brain syndrome is associated with the loss or dysfunction of brain cells or any neurological degeneration of unknown origin. The terms are also thought to be synonymous (Goldfarb 1974; Birren et al. 1956). "Senility and organic brain syndrome can be used interchangeably. They mean the same thing" (psychiatrist, GST). Choice of terminology reflects conventions of the institution rather than discrimination between the two possible diseases.

The mental health practitioner employs both individual and standardized criteria in making a diagnosis. As might be expected, individual criteria are variable and sometimes in conflict with conventional clinical judgments.

> The psychotic has systematic delusions which usually have an "olfactory"-flavor. (psychiatric resident 1, CSH)

> I don't use the textbook on diagnostic characteristics. You need to go with the situation. I've a general sense of what psychosis is, and on the basis of general questions, can draw a picture of psychosis. I look for the range of normal behavior, and behavior which goes beyond that. (social worker, GST)

> Delusions associated with old age are equivalent to senility. (psychiatric nurse 8, CSH)

The mental status exam is the standardized measure; in fact, organic brain syndrome is defined clinically in terms of poor performance on the exam.

Organic brain syndrome is characterized by disorientation for time, place and person; memory loss, both remote and recent; deficits of general information of the simplest kind; and inability to do even simple calculations. Defects of grasp and comprehension and also impaired judgment, as well as shallowness and lability of affect, are often but not invariably present. (Goldfarb 1974)

Cited below are the categories and commonly used test questions:

Orientation to time, place, person
   Where are you?
   What is your name?
   What is the date today?
Memory
   Who is the President of the United States?
   I'm going to tell you three words, "red barn," "banana," "Chevrolet." I want you to remember them because I'm going to ask you later on.
Symbolic process
   "The proverb test is the more sophisticated exam" (psychiatric nurse 8, CSH).
   What does it mean, "People who live in glass houses shouldn't throw rocks"?
   What does it mean, "A rolling stone gathers no moss"?
Calculations
   Count backward from 100 by 7s.
Form test (occasionally used)
   I'm going to draw a figure, then you draw the same thing.

On the basis of these standardized questions, supplemented by individual criteria, the mental health examiner determines the presence of decline, deficit, and disease in organic matter, brain cells, and neurons.

The syndrome (measured by the mental status exam) is presumptive evidence of brain cell loss or dysfunction. (Goldfarb 1974)

The form test is one of the first indicators of senile brain disease. It indicates a loss of cortical brain cells. (psychiatrist 2, CH)

The judgment is a matter of inference rather than direct observation. Since it seems unlikely that confusion causes brain cell deterioration, it is accepted that deterioration causes confusion. Some researchers argue that there is quantifiable corroboration of the correlation between the extent of a cell loss and behavior:

Early in the process little change may be seen in the brain or in behavior. As cell loss becomes more marked, the patient begins to have difficulties in his everyday functioning which usually give rise to personal, family and community problems. (Goldfarb 1974)

In practice, however, there is no direct empirical measurement of the organic impairment on a case-by-case basis. Other researchers challenge the validity of even the correlation.

> ... no good correlation exists between the degree, distribution, and characters of various abnormal changes and the age and state of the neuro-function of the individual (Wolf 1959)

> Interviewer: Is there a correlation between degree of confusion and degree of brain deterioration?
> Psychiatrist (GST): No.

Still others argue that organic deterioration does not independently cause confusion. Deterioration acts in association with other variables: "Just knowing the degree of organic deficit doesn't tell you much. You must also look at such things as environment" (geriatric psychiatrist).

The mental status exam plays a minor and perfunctory part in intake evaluations on nonelderly. In some cases, the results of a mental status exam in an initial evaluation are not even reported to the admission team. Instead, the evaluator examines in detail the recent events in the candidate's life. Often the confused elderly who appear at Central State Hospital are poor informants about themselves. If they arrive unaccompanied, there is no information available about daily life performance. The hospital staff does not search out independent documentation by going to the neighborhood or residence. The staff also complains about inadequate information with nursing home referrals. It appears that the mental status exam is, in part, an expedient substitute for the lack of more useful information that the evaluator is either unwilling or unable to ascertain.

It is not uncommon to find multiple diagnoses because single traits are symptomatic of more than one diagnostic category. Therefore, one category clinically appears (or "presents") much like another.

> Her final diagnosis was, organic dementia, psychosis with etiology unknown, possible schizophrenic depression. (social worker 1, GST; psychiatric resident 8, CSH)

> Even though the senile and the psychotics present the same, they're very different diseases. (psychiatric resident 7, CSH)

As a last resort, mental health professionals use ex post facto or "pudding" variables to make a definitive diagnosis. The elderly patient's response or lack of response to speculative treatments defines the nature of the pathology:

The proof is in the pudding. If you give a patient antipsychotic medication, and he gets better, then you know he was psychotic. (social worker 1, GST)

The only way you can make the diagnosis is to try different medication treatments. The treatment that works tells you what was wrong. (psychiatric nurse 1, GST)

Interviewer: How do you distinguish senility from depression?
Psychiatric nurse 8: Depression is a whole different illness. You use antidepressants and ECT.

In spite of the uncertainties and subtleties in clinical evaluation, the professionals are usually certain of the accuracy of their diagnostic conclusions.

It's not difficult to tell the difference between senile confusion and psychosis. (psychiatric resident 1, CSH)

Usually you can tell right away. (psychiatric nurse 7, CSH)

Such certitude, however, seems unwarranted in the face of confusion about the definitions, etiology, and clinical manifestations. The evaluator's confidence is more closely related to opinions about the aging process than to diagnostic ability.

(Evaluating a wanderer on whom the practitioner has no history at all): He wouldn't be a candidate for psych because he's organic not functional. It's not reversible. Some of it might be. I don't know that much about him. (psychiatric nurse 6, CSH)

Senility is just aging. It happens to everyone. Old people who are confused are just getting senile. (psychiatric resident 1, CSH)

People who are old and worn out are called senile. The aging process has just caught up with them. (psychiatric nurse 7, CSH)

To recapitulate, Claiborne mental health evaluators made the following arguments in defense of their diagnostic confidence:

(1) The problem is that inexperienced and untrained practitioners make inaccurate diagnoses. (2) The science of diagnosing senility is not well defined. Advancements do not occur because there's no treatment incentive. If the mental health clinician diagnoses senility, it means do not intervene; if he diagnoses no senility, it means do not intervene. Clinicians can accu-

rately diagnose senility if they are cautious and thorough. That means taking the environment into account. (geriatric psychiatrist)

The combined effect of professional confidence and diagnostic confusion leaves confused elderly with little opportunity to defend themselves against the hopelessness of the diagnosis: "There's very little in the intake evaluation that provides definitive evidence of treatability" (psychiatrist 1, PH). Important variables, such as acute onset of confusion (see Chapter 9 for an elaboration) or successful self-maintenance in the community, may not appear at the time of evaluation. Basic a priori assumptions about the presence of organic brain deterioration further discourages the search for alternative explanations. Even the elderly who pass the mental status exam and maintain conventional lifestyles may receive the same senile dementia diagnosis with the psychiatric qualification: "She's in the early stages of her disease" (psychiatric resident 9, CSH).

Evidence of prior pathology does alter the usual diagnostic conclusions. For example, youthful patients who have grown old in the hospital become "burned-out schizophrenics" rather than "senile." Similarly, aged drinkers are given an alternative label: "We see a lot of old alcoholics. When an old man comes in whose behavior is bizarre, he's drunk not crazy" (welfare worker 4, CH). An elderly gentleman on the inpatient service with "extensive peripheral arteriodisease" was not diagnosed organic brain syndrome because the consulting family psychiatrist and staff social worker were interested in his "family problem." Labeling him senile would only interfere with his social utility to those interested in family problems, even though the correlation between senility and arteriodisease is taken for granted. He is also tidy, well-mannered, and passive, and therefore totally unobjectionable as a ward patient.

Negotiationg the Admission Decision

In addition to the clinical evaluation of pathology, the admission decision is the result of candidate/evaluator negotiations and external community and organizational pressures. When their ideas about a desirable outcome differ, the hospital's admitting officer and the individual applicant may enter into protracted negotiations.

[An elderly man requested admission.] We offered him admission to the day hospital, but he refused it. He was here from 9:00 to 5:00. We kept running into him in the hallway. We'd make other offers which he refused. Finally at 5:00, he took the name and number of an adult crash pad, and left. I never heard from him again. (psychiatric resident 10, CSH)

In general, the hospital has the superior bargaining position, as is illustrated in the above quote. However, the applicant with a reciprocal service to offer the evaluator is in a better position, and the outcome of negotiations is more likely to favor the applicant's preferences.

> [The resident explained that the elderly lady with "advanced dementia" had "overextended" herself with community involvement. She needed to be less involved.]
>
> Psychiatric resident 10: She's a major community resource! She could help me place my patients, so I offered her a job.
>
> Continuing care worker 1: Is that what she really needs—another job?
>
> Psychiatric resident 10: Well, it's a barter. I help her, and she helps me.

Given the resident's evaluation, it is not obvious who got the better deal. While his analysis and decision conflict, the lady did obtain the assistance she wanted in spite of her "advanced dementia" diagnosis. When the situation is reversed, and the hospital wants to admit a person who refuses to acknowledge his or her potential candidacy, their differences may also be negotiated. Again, the hospital-designated candidate has the inferior negotiating position. The candidate can be involuntarily committed over all protestations.*

> When we got her [an elderly lady] to the hospital, she began to struggle furiously. She pointed her finger at me, and said, "You were once my girl. If you take me out of my home, I'll die!" She's now on the service, and is doing fine. But you never know how a case will turn out. (psychiatric nurse 2, GST)

The various admission labels† applied to prospective patients do leave some room for maneuvering. Those who refuse voluntary admission may be offered conditional voluntary admission as an alternative to commitment.

---

*This is an emotionally and politically sensitive encounter and one that professionals prefer to confront inside the hospital rather than in the community. In one case, the psychiatric resident duped his candidate patient in order to get her inside the hospital: "The neighbors called the hospital to complain, and I went out to her house. She was psychotic so I admitted her. I convinced her to come to the hospital for an evaluation, and she was committed" (psychiatric resident 11, CSH).

†The patient enters the hospital as either a voluntary or involuntary (committed) admission. A voluntary admission can be either conditional or nonconditional. If it is conditional, the patient agrees not to leave the hospital without giving a three-day notice. An involuntary admission can be limited to ten days (referred to as being "sectioned" or coming in on a "pink paper") or can be court-committed, which applies to the "criminally insane." The term "committed" is rarely used.

> Fortunately I was able to convince her to go with me in a taxi to the hospital. I told her, "Either sign a 'voluntary' or we are going to commit you." Once they understand their situation, only the really psychotic will refuse. (psychiatric nurse 2, GST)

As a representative of the hospital, the admitting officer must take the needs of the institution into account. Old people, also, have institutional affiliations; they rarely come to the hospital alone or without referral. Referrals might come from the Visiting Nurse Association, the geriatric outreach worker, the police, a community health clinic, a neighbor, family member, or nursing home. The majority come from nursing homes. In essence, the hospital must service the referring station as well as the prospective patient. In the following illustrations, admission is not determined by patient characteristics, but by nursing home and community pressure.

> The nursing home staff had given her more and more time until she used them up. They said she hobbled across her room on a broken leg and tried to jump out the window. They brought her here. She was not really psychotic, so we didn't get into psychodynamics with her. In this case we are not treating her so much as manipulating the social response. (psychiatric resident 2, CSH)

> She was against admission but the community wanted her in, so we had to "section" [commit] her, and have her brought in by the police. (psychiatric nurse 1, CSH)

> She has been getting worse—wandering around at two A.M., and rummaging through the trash. The people downstairs in her building say she throws furniture at night and wakes up the infant. There is neighborhood pressure to get her out. (psychiatric nurse 2, GST)

To summarize, admission has been discussed as an organizational function, as the institutional analogue to diagnosis, and as a social process. The admission mechanism affords an organization control over the boundaries of its patient domain. With respect to confused elderly who are usually regarded as undesirable patients, controlling admission is essential to the hospital. Admission decisions are supposedly based on professional judgments of mental impairment. From a diagnostician's point of view, the mental status exam is the standardized test for senility and therefore the principal determinant. Other factors, however, were observed to play a significant part. The use of ex post facto and multiple diagnoses and the inferential uncertainty of the mental status exam point to a lack of technical precision and sophistication in diagnosing senility. Admitting or rejecting the candidate is obviously influenced by more than ambiguous diagnosis. In fact, admission decisions are a negotiated social process. Outcome is determined by the bargaining strengths of admitting officers, candidates, and other community stations with vested interests.

THE INPATIENT SERVICE

The inpatient service at Central State Hospital was recently "unitized." That is, adult and adolescent patients admitted to the hospital service are assigned to one of three wards according to their place of residence. Therefore, all Claiborne residents, including the elderly, are admitted to "Service A." Life on Service A for the geriatric patient is influenced by the tone of the ward and its physical amenities. The staff's expectations for these patients profoundly affect their status and relations among ward peers. Discharge from the service is determined not only by the patient's performance but by the hospital's organizational alliances.

Conditions on the Ward

Service A is administrated by the supervising psychiatrist and the chief resident, a third-year psychiatric resident. Ward staff, nurses, social workers, and attendants, are organized in six teams led by first-year psychiatric residents. Patient population ranges from 25 to 30, and each patient is assigned to a specific psychiatric resident and team. Nurses and attendants are primarily responsible for day-to-day maintenance of the ward.

There is a consensus among hospital staff that the hospital building itself is deteriorated and ill-equipped.

The hospital's in bad shape. It's really shabby. (executive administrator, CSH)

One reason I never want to be a patient here is because of the physical setup. We're so ill-equipped. (psychiatric nurse 10, CSH)

The appearance of Service A is unappealing. The walls are painted in army green and grey. The paint is filthy and peeling. The community room windows look out onto the exterior wall of adjoining hospital wings. The room is lined with ragged, sometimes cushionless couches. On an average day, breakfast dishes, trays, and leftover food are left on tables, chairs, and the floor until noon, when they are collected, and lunch is served. The remains of lunch are left lying about until dinner time. This provides some patients, usually the elderly, with an opportunity to go picking among the leftovers throughout the day.

The service is as ill-equipped as it is unattractive. For example, there are two major toilet facilities, one in each wing. In one, four sinks stand along the wall. There is a mirror above one of the sinks; the other three mirrors have been removed. There are no towels, soap, or toilet paper. "If I want to wash before I go to bed, I have to hunt and hunt for even a tiny chip of soap. And I'm afraid to wash my feet. It's so dirty, I'm afraid of getting some foot disease" (Simon, patient).

There is one washing machine, but no dryer. Patients must hang their laundry on a rack to dry and hope their clothes are still there when they return.

The prevailing tone is one of disorder and confusion. The staff and patients struggle together to make the ward habitable. The staff focuses on controlling deviant behavior and the patients focus on daily custodial maintenance. A large part of staff meeting time is devoted to clarifying and modifying restrictions and privileges. On the ward, the staff-patient encounters are peacekeeping rather than therapeutic exercises.

> We're so busy. All we have time for is management. (psychiatric nurse 2, CSH)

> We spend a lot of time just being sure patients don't break regulations [general rules] and restrictions [individual rules]. The staff calls it "setting limits." (attendant, CSH)

The weekly "community meeting" was the primary forum for patients to organize and lobby for more supplies, a cleaner ward, protection of personal property, better food, and so on.

There were occasions when the service became so disordered that ward performance broke down, and nothing worked. In Goffman's terms the patients as audience refused to support the show (1959). Instead, they complained and confronted the staff with its inconsistencies.

> [After the chief resident asked for the opinion of the patients] Do you think the staff really listens to what we have to say, or is it cooption and mutual masturbation? (Linda, patient)

> They only have time to enforce the rules. They don't have time to listen to us. (Carl, patient)

> We need to clean up this ward, and I think the staff should help us. Or are they too good? (Peter, patient)

When staff and patients tacitly agree to carry on in the face of inconsistencies, the effect on ward performance is just as damaging. During a community meeting, the patients discussed purchasing a coffee pot with patient funds. At the same time, there were sounds of a struggle in the background. One by one, staff persons filtered out of the meeting to participate in the confrontation somewhere down the hallway, behind closed doors. The appearance of business as usual and the staff-patient dialogue were socially contaminated.

There is universal recognition by staff and patients that conditions on the ward create an intolerable tension.* The chief resident talked about the "restlessness" of patients.

> It was tense this weekend. I thought all hell was going to break loose, but we made it. (attendant 1, CSH)

> This place is out of control. One guy played his radio until midnight because the attendants are afraid of him. They wouldn't come in and turn it down. They were hiding in the nurses' station. (Simon, patient)

Ward Society and the Elderly Patient

The problems of chaos and disorder are attributed, in part, to the presence of the elderly on the service:

> Psychiatric nurse 2: The bedrooms are an eyesore. Less than half the beds are made at any one time.
> Claire [patient]: But Margie comes in and tears up the beds after they're made.
> Psychiatric nurse 2: Yes, she does do that. If you would direct her out of the rooms, it would help a lot.
> Claire: We do that, but it happens anyway.
> Ralph [patient]: Look, here comes "Miss Linen" now. [Margie passed through the room carrying bed sheets.]

> You can't keep anything in your drawers. The crazy old people are always going through them. (Peter, patient)

> Allen [an elderly patient] comes in during the night, shits right by my bed, then goes through the drawers. And where's the attendant? Hiding in the nurses' station. (Paul, patient)

---

*The statements of past employees on the same service document the presence of similar circumstances in previous years.

> I had to leave. The pressure just got to be too much for me. I'm much happier here in the outpatient department. (psychiatric nurse 5, CSH)

> When they asked me to stay, I agreed only if they'd take me off the ward. (psychiatric nurse 3, CSH)

The staff actively opposes the placement of the elderly on their ward. Their rationales assert concern for the welfare of the elderly as well as the difficulties of dealing with the elderly.

> The most obnoxious behavior is the elderly defecating all over the place. That's much worse than even physical struggles with patients. (psychiatric nurse 3, CSH)

> We don't have the proper physical supports like bannisters or handles on the toilet walls. (chief resident, CSH)

> An adult ward is not a good place for the elderly. It's dangerous for them. They're vulnerable to attack by adolescents who see them as weak parent figures, and turn their hostility towards them. Beyond that, they tend to get run over in the crush of daily life. (chief resident, CSH)

The staff does not expect any improvement in their mental status, and management is a misuse of manpower.

> They consume a great deal of staff time just for custodial care. (psychiatric nurse 9, CSH)

> For a ward administrator, Margie is a real pain in the ass. She takes a lot of time and staff resources. (chief resident, CSH)

The elderly do not participate in any therapeutic regimens. Their days are marked by inactivity and restless wandering. Treatment consists of passive tolerance for their disruptions. When daily routine necessitates encounters—meals, medication rounds, and blood pressure checks—the staff is gentle and polite.

> While she was on the service, she was treated like any other old person. She just did a lot of sitting around. (attendant 2, CSH)

> We work with her a lot—comb her hair, the person administering drugs talks to her. We've tried placing her several times. (social worker 3, CSH)

> An elderly lady sat in the same chair every day. With one exception, the 10:45 medication rounds, no one spoke to her between breakfast and lunch. (observation)

The elderly person on the ward becomes the mental patients' mental patient. Their uniquely deviant behavior segregates them from the other patients. As mentioned before, the others complain about the elderly stealing linen, hoarding toilet paper, and picking through trash. They are repulsed by the elderly's failure to show proper middle-class disdain for garbage. The staff and general patient population commiserate together over the "geriatric problem." Professionals encourage patients to be tolerant and have pity because "She's demented. There's nothing we can do for her" (chief resident, CSH). The younger mental patients accept this definition of the situation:

> She's just an old lady, and doesn't know any better. (Harriet, patient)

> You have to be careful around Margie. She'll reach out and pull your hair or grab your clothes. But she can't help it. She doesn't know any better. (ex-mental hospital patient)

The staff and patients exhibit their low expectations of the elderly by being impressed with any show of their competence: "Margie signed a get-well card for the custodian. The staff and patients were all startled, and were curious to see her signature. She was congratulated by everyone" (observation).

Patient solidarity and fraternalization are important reorganizing influences of the hospital (Goffman 1961). Patients are united by their common struggle against the institution: "Being at Central State has been a good thing. Most important are the 'wardships' I've formed while a patient here" (Peter, patient). The elderly suffer the same disadvantages as the other patients on the ward. In spite of their mutual burdens and hardships of the situation, the elderly are excluded from this fraternalization because of their low status in ward society.

They are also scapegoats. The service has a ready explanation for disorder and missing property.

> This place wouldn't look so bad if the old people didn't create such disorder. (social worker 1, CSH)

> Chief resident: You have to put your things away or the old people will walk off with them.
> Matthew [patient]: They're not the only ones. There are some who steal.

Getting off the ward is a privilege granted to the most reliable patients. Because the elderly are thought to be too confused or too physically infirm, they rarely share in patient activities outside the ward. Their total confinement and visibility exceed those of all other patients.

Survival Strategies

Maintaining security and dignity is a problem for all the hospital patients. In response to confinement on the ward, even the most confused of the geriatric patients employ survival tactics and face-saving gestures. Conformity and resignation characterize the struggle of some elderly to survive in a disordered and oppressive atmosphere. Their techniques are

Tactful silence: When the staff discussed Simon, an elderly patient, they agreed that he was "uncommunicative, but doing pretty well. He doesn't have any complaints." After Simon assured himself that I was not a staff member, he vigorously complained to me about the noise, chaos, and disorganization. He called the hospital "a zoo," and the community meeting "a joke." He was extremely unhappy with his situation. (observation)

Graciousness: She may cause a lot of trouble, but she can be very charming in comparison to some of them. (attendant 3, CSH)

Calculated caution [In response to a loud threatening exchange between two male patients, Cassandra, an elderly lady, said]: I don't mix in their affairs; best just to keep out of it.

Cassandra sits in the same place every day. Her spot is as safe or safer than any place on the ward. It is the only place [near the front door] where a staff person is always present. (observation)

Selective perception: Interviewer [to an elderly lady who is hard of hearing]: Does it bother you not being able to hear what's happening on the ward? Lady: Oh, no! In fact it's an advantage here because you don't hear all the commotion.

In contrast, other elderly refuse to acknowledge, and oppose the professional's definition of their situation. Their tactics are

Redefinition: Of course, I'm not mental, thank the Lord. If I remain here much longer, though, I'll be stark raving mad and then I'll have reason for staying. Last week I became ill with all the noise, shouting, screaming, and what not. There must be some way out of this mess. I can't afford to have a real breakdown. (Betty, patient)

This place is worse than Russia. They've got me locked up with a bunch of nuts. (Frank, patient)

Manipulation: In less than one week on the ward, she'd written a letter to the executive director complaining about her treatment. When he came on the floor to investigate, the staff was in an uproar. (psychology intern, CSH)

She's whipping up her family with outrageous stories about what happens on the service. (psychiatrist, Service A, CSH)

Politicking [During a community meeting, Lisa, an elderly lady, denounced the service, and threatened]: I'm going to sue for damages done to my mental well-being, and I encourage the rest of the patients to join me.

Comic relief [Frank, an elderly patient, had an infected foot. This was a real handicap for the most notorious wanderer on the ward. It was impossible to keep him confined. On one occasion when he was up and about, a nurse challenged him]: What are you doing? Frank: I'm exercising my foot.

The hospitalized elderly, however, lack the professional authority and status to define social realities (Wiseman 1970). Their gestures of protest become further evidence of confusion. For example, "Her overt independence is probably a screen for emotional dependence" (psychiatrist, Service A, CSH). A dinner invitation was transformed into documentation of mental illness. Betty, an elderly patient, wrote a letter to the psychology intern's wife. This letter is now part of her medical record. . . . he most certainly is brilliant and has such a future in his profession. I have met psychiatrists since 1961, and I consider myself an authority on the subject. . . . Hoping to have you and your husband over for dinner soon, I remain, Very respectfully yours. . . .

LENGTH OF STAY, PLACEMENT, AND FOLLOW-UP

The length of a patient's stay in the hospital depends on ward behavior, financing, and placement resources. In spite of the mental hospital's contemporary self-definition as an acute care setting, it is more difficult for most patients to obtain discharge than admission (Rosenhan 1973). Eligibility for discharge is determined by evidence of improvement. In general, "improvement" implies conformity to house rules and adherence to personal restrictions. The patient is "doing better" when

. . . she's very "appropriate," keeping restrictions to the "t." . . . she smokes only in the dayroom now. . . . he showered, washed his hair and clothes. . . . he helped with [food] trays. . . . she took her medication. . . . her language has improved. . . . she's no longer assaultive. . . . she's expressing sadness about termination of staff. . . . he isn't panhandling and going back to his room any more.

Given the ward environment, it is not surprising that keeping clean and being orderly are important to the staff. The simplified ward society offers few other options to patients for demonstrating sanity. Because the elderly are poor performers on these variables, they have even less opportunity to demonstrate improvement.

Fidelity to staff expectations is rewarded with a progression of freedoms, called privileges. Discharge is the ultimate privilege. From total restriction to discharge, the possible variations are seclusion with patient stripped and locked in; seclusion with the door opened; restricted to common room; restricted to common room and dayroom; full service—the patient can go anywhere on the floor; group to meals (or pool or gym)—the patient can accompany supervised group outings; full hospital—the patient can wander through the building; hours out—the patient can leave the hospital for a specified amount of time; overnight; weekend pass; discharge.

When the service staff wants to discharge an elderly patient, evidence of "stability" replaces improvement as an essential criterion. Stability, measured by the absence of overt disruptive behavior, implies an adjustment in medication.

> We originally tried to send him home with medication. (social worker 2, CSH)

> We started Lisa on Lithium because of a history of manic depression. She became Lithium toxic. Then we put her on Haldol, and sent her to a nursing home. (psychiatric nurse 1, CSH)

> She wasn't getting any better so we put her on Tyndol and placed her. (psychiatric nurse 1, CSH)

The service staff rarely returns elderly patients to their own homes or families. Between January and June 1974, only three of the sixteen elderly patients discharged from Central State went home (Central State Hospital statistics). In the absence of independent wealth, the elderly cannot be discharged to a nursing home until federal or state financing has been cleared. Applications for federal and state financing can be delayed through inaction or rejection.

> It's necessary to file for Medicaid and SSI simultaneously even though SSI automatically qualifies the recipient for Medicaid. SSI takes two or three months to get cleared, and we just don't have that much time. (continuing care worker 1, CSH)

> You never know for sure what action will be taken on your application. No qualification decision can be made locally. They're all sent to Baltimore, and the national headquarters has a quota for rejections. So you never know what will become of your application. (continuing care worker 1, CSH)

When financing problems cannot be immediately resolved, the patient waits in the hospital. One elderly lady has been in the hospital for two years. Her continued presence is attributed solely to financing problems. Psychiatric nurse 3 described her as the "sanest person on the service." Her problems are complicated by her own refusal to cooperate.

> Her problem is she has too much money to be eligible for Medicaid. She won't spend any of it, so welfare won't pay for nursing home placement. The

court appointed a guardian six months ago to locate money and pay her bills. He's been farting around. Eight months ago we contacted Social Security about her checks and change of address. We have yet to hear from them. (social worker 2, CSH)*

There are two elderly patients on the service who have failed so many placements that they will stay in the hospital until they die. Their behavior is so disorderly that no nursing home will keep them. The hospital staff decided that attempting another placement would be a disservice to the patients since they would inevitably return.

He hits and bites. No nursing home will accept that. He'll be here until he dies. (chief resident, CSH)

We tolerate him. Nursing homes don't or can't. We made a decision to let him stay here. (social worker 2, CSH)

There is, of course, great interest in all opportunities to discharge chronic geriatric patients. Like all other patient care decisions, however, placement is described as a professionally evaluated therapeutic action. The result is wide discrepancies between the description and the practice.

Ideal: We place patients according to the nature of their problems, and the willingness and ability of the home. (chief resident, CSH)

Actual: . . . it was a quick transfer. (social worker 1, CSH)

. . . a shot in the dark. He made such a nuisance of himself people really wanted him out. (social worker 2, CSH)

The institutions have a blacklist of homes they never use. If Central State has a really troublesome patient, they'll use these homes. Their rationale is that these are the only homes that will take them. There's also a kind of revenge in getting even with those patients who have given the staff a hard time. (welfare worker 4)

Ideal: We have a new policy. We now take patients to the potential nursing home placement for a visit. The patient sees the home, and the nursing home staff sees the patient. (psychiatric nurse 3, CSH)

---

*For two years, the welfare liaison worker has refused to approve the application because the lady is suspected of having money in a bank. During this time, her situation actually has become more complicated since she was not receiving her Social Security checks. Those accumulated earnings must also be collected and spent. The welfare worker and staff suspect she has $8,000 saved. Since welfare rate is $1,400 for 30 days, the lady has "spent" her savings, and public financing will be approved once the money is turned over to the state.

Actual: We're dragging some of these old people to the nursing home. We shove them out our door. If a nursing home is willing to work with them, and they say they will accept them, then we'll send them. (psychiatric nurse 3, CSH)

Ideal: We always return a patient to the home he came from, or we always try to. (chief resident, CSH)

Actual: A nursing home patient discharged to the mental hospital has usually caused so much trouble that the embittered staff refuses to reaccept the patient. (continuing care worker 2, CSH)

A nursing home is not always "selected" by the placement staff. Often the home notifies the hospital of an empty bed, and the service discharges its most troublesome patient.

The elderly most likely to go when a placement becomes available are those who have caused the most trouble on the service. (social worker 1, CSH)

The Hunt Nursing Home called a few weeks back saying they had three beds. It's easy to understand that we immediately had three people ready to place. (psychiatric nurse 1, GST)

The willingness of the hospital to use knowingly homes they consider to be hazardous was apparent in the geriatric specialists' team discussion of a nursing home where an ex-patient died (see Chapter 6). When an elderly lady was readmitted to Service A, she complained vociferously about physical abuse in a nursing home. The staff was already familiar with the problem in that home. Its only response was: "I don't think she was ever beaten up, but she certainly saw it happen, and was threatened herself" (psychiatric nurse 3, CSH).

Placement in nursing homes is particularly traumatic for the patients who have never lived in nursing homes before.

We placed two really bad people in that home. Both were first-timers. One who'd been committed wanted to go back to her apartment. She had a terrible time for three weeks. We were always going out there. The other was an old man who became assaultive, and his wife didn't want him around anymore. (psychiatric nurse 3, CSH)

The staff is sometimes faced with "cooling-out" the patient. In at least one case, a patient was not informed of her fate until the placement had been completed. While transition was bureaucratically smoothed by deliberately concealing information from the patient, the hospital merely shifted the burden to the home and jeopardized patient adjustment: "The nursing home called because no one told the lady she would not be going home. She still has plans to return to her apartment. They're worried, and want us to come out and tell her" (psychiatric nurse 1, GST).

Regardless of their original residence, some elderly refuse to cooperate with the staff's placement plans. An elderly patient's resistance is not accepted as evidence that placement is premature or countertherapeutic. The staff would rather coerce the patient physically than miss a placement opportunity.

> She went out for a nursing home visit. She didn't like the place but they liked her. When the day came for her to leave, she refused to put on her coat. We put her shoes on, and she kicked them off. We tried to tie her to a wheelchair, but she was too big. We argued with her, "There's nothing more we can do for you. If we have to carry you out, you'll disgrace yourself." After we carried her as far as the lobby, she walked the rest of the way. (psychology intern, CSH)

The notion of community follow-up for a patient discharged from the hospital service is central to community mental health doctrine. The state department of mental health requires the hospital to contact every ex-patient at least four times in the first year after discharge. The staff claims to adhere conscientiously to follow-up doctrine: "We have a 'leaning out' policy. The first week out of the hospital and into a nursing home, we visit several times, gradually withdrawing completely" (chief resident, CSH). When follow-up prevents frequent readmission, the hospital and the ex-patient are beneficiaries: "If we don't do follow-up, we have a greater placement problem with more frequent readmissions and outraged nursing home directors who refuse to accept any more of our patients" (chief resident, CSH).

A large proportion of the community visits are responses to requests from nursing homes. The ex-patient's satisfaction or dissatisfaction with placement is independent of follow-up unless it results in disruptive behavior. In this respect, a hospital's community visit is similar in function to the geriatric specialist's nursing home consultation for disruptive patients: "Our approach on the community visit is to tell the staff about the patient's brilliant past, counsel them to have patience, and compliment their efforts. Obviously our focus is not on change, but tolerance" (psychology intern, CSH).

Even though the usefulness of follow-up is widely acknowledged, it is rarely practiced with discharged elderly. Studies show geropsychiatric ex-patients do not receive the additional care they need. For example, Elizabeth Markson and co-workers (1973) found that out of 111 geropsychiatric patients discharged from a mental hospital, 50 percent were in need of psychiatric outpatient care, forty percent were in need of medical care, and 22 percent in need of supervision at home. On Service A, community visits are infrequent (but made more often than on the other services).

> This last year I was to oversee follow-up care, so I know not much was done. Maybe one community visit a week was made by the staff. I sometimes went twice a week. (psychiatric nurse 3, CSH)

> My neighbor was admitted to Central State. She was there two weeks, and discharged home. I went over to see them about her. They said there was nothing they could do so they gave her Tyndol, and sent her home. In their records, they'd written, "No plans for follow-up." It's really crazy. (psychiatric nurse 1, CH)

In fact, community visits even once a week are considered to be exceptionally frequent. Such solicitousness is reserved for the special interest elderly patient: "Last time he was placed we made a real effort to follow. Visits were made once a week" (occupational therapist, CSH).

In addition to follow-up visits, an aftercare program is supposedly sent with the patient to the nursing home. This, too, is neglected.

> The law requires a follow-up plan to be written in the discharge. Well, it just isn't done. Patients leave without any written aftercare program. And the nursing homes don't ask for one either. (continuing care worker 1, CSH)

> Some of the proper things happen once in awhile, but it's inconsistent and disorganized. (continuing care worker 1, CSH)

The service's failure to make community visits and write aftercare plans is consistent with the hospital's psychoanalytic rather than community orientation. The elderly supposedly are beyond rehabilitation, therefore, a serious aftercare program is unnecessary. Follow-up is only useful when it protects the service from readmission. Ward conditions and staff perspectives also limit community follow-up. The reluctance of psychiatric residents to go into nursing homes has already been discussed. Only attendants and psychiatric nurses make community visits on a routine basis. The service staff, which is most engrossed in daily management of the ward, is also responsible for community follow-up. Under present conditions, ward management is so demanding that responsibilities off the floor have low priority.

> Those people on top of the staff hierarchy don't do many community visits, so it's left to us. And it's difficult for us because we're so tied up with ward routine and management. (psychiatric nurse 3, CSH)

> I had to schedule this visit for a time after I get off work. We just don't have time to leave during work hours. (psychiatric nurse 2, CSH)

STABILIZING TREATMENTS

Most of the elderly who come or are brought to the hospital door are turned away (referred elsewhere) for reasons already discussed. There are exceptions; emergencies, outside pressure, and chronic patients force encounters with the hospital staff. The hospital has a preestablished assortment of treatments, and its responses are confined to these guidelines. Usually the notion of treatment identifies some professionally prescribed action intended to improve the patient's condition by reducing pathology. It is also agreed, however, that senility is an irreversible pathology. Therefore, the treatments at the hospital staff's disposal are redefined as stabilization strategies instead of rehabilitation strategies.

The staff has a highly generalized definition of treatment. Blood pressure and temperature checks are part of the daily treatment regime for hospitalized elderly. Discharge itself is described as a treatment: "We've tried everything with her—one-to-one, behavior mod, different meds, ECT, OT—we've even tried nursing home placement several times" (social worker 3, CSH). Since confused elderly do not qualify for more esoteric intervention, "treatment" becomes any hospital activity that engages them.

Medication and Hospitalization

Elderly patients are stabilized by "correcting" their medication. It is assumed that a troublesome geriatric patient has been improperly (or inadequately) medicated. Such corrections may be first attempted in the nursing home by the Geriatric Specialist Team (see Chapter 6) and ward staff who follow up at the home's request: "If we intervene early enough, we can manage the patient, that is, regulate his meds, in the home. Otherwise it's done in the hospital" (psychiatric resident 1, CSH). If the home's patience is spent, and the medication adjustment fails, then the patient is admitted to the hospital in order to stabilize.

We admitted her so we can regulate her meds. (psychiatric nurse 3, CSH)

Monitoring, that's the whole issue. (psychology intern, CSH)

By offering stabilization as a special form of treatment, mental health doctrine attributes therapeutic qualities to the use of tranquilizing drugs. In fact, their use is a pragmatic compromise with environmental needs. On the inpatient service, tranquilization was equated with security and used as a matter of convenience or as a substitute for manpower. Conditions in the environment, not individual behavior, were critical factors.

Attendant: He's refusing to take his meds.

Psychiatric resident 5: He can't stay if he isn't going to take his medications. He can't get special privileges. If he stays, he must take his meds. *That's our only insurance.* We have only two choices—medicate him or discharge him.

On Mellaril, Katie became less cantankerous and settled down. The difference was, on Mellaril you could nag her, and she'd eventually take a shower. Without Mellaril, if you nagged her, she'd hit. (psychiatric nurse 1, CSH)

If Margie gets her PRN, it's almost always in the evening because she's harder to control at night when there are fewer staff on duty. (psychiatric nurse 1, CSH)

Equating medication with treatment is complicated further by the mental health specialists' criticism of its use with the elderly and by the uncertainty in its application.

Medication is the last thing to think about. (psychiatrist, GST)

Medication creates more problems than it solves because of side effects, but the general approach is, if you have a problem, medicate it. (psychiatric resident 1, CSH)

Simon was on Elavil but he grew toxic. We were afraid he'd arrest any minute. (psychiatric nurse 1, CSH)

Within the mental health profession there is disagreement about the selection of the proper psychoactive drug for use with elderly. For example

Thorazine: Thorazine is too strong for old people, but Haldol works wonders (psychiatric nurse 1, CH)

The psychiatrist recommended a change in medication to Thorazine. He says he's had some luck with that. (psychiatric nurse 2, PH)

Elavil: Simon and Lisa were on Elavil. (psychiatric nurse 1, CSH)

Never give anyone over 65 Elavil. It drops their blood pressure too much. (psychology intern, CSH)

Finally, community agents outside the hospital are openly critical of the "correcting" medication policy. From their point of view, "correcting" means increasing the tranquilizer dosage, and the effect is to displace the problem rather than resolve it.

They [CSH] use massive doses of drugs. If I order 25 mg., they'd order 200. I always use the least, not the most. (private physician 1, house doctor, Court Nursing Home)

When an old person is in the hospital, he gets massive does of tranquilizers. The sedated patient returns to the nursing home. The house doctors don't use heavy dosages. They write new, reduced medication orders. The patient acts up, and is returned to the hospital where his medication is once again increased. The cycle begins again. (welfare worker 3)

Electroconvulsive Therapy (ECT)

Although electroconvulsive therapy (ECT) is not a "curative" procedure, according to the Central State Hospital ECT Manual, it is, nonetheless, a form of therapy (as the name implies).

Outside of surgery, this is the one medical treatment where you see immediate results. (psychiatric resident 5, CSH)

I think he's treatable. You can work with this guy. I'd recommend ECT. (psychiatrist, GST)

Outpatient ECT may restore a patient to functioning without necessitating hospitalization. As such, it constitutes an important community mental health treatment modality: efficient, inexpensive, available. (CSH ECT Manual)

In the past it has been criticized as barbaric, a means for vindictive staff to pacify troublesome patients. It is increasingly popular, however, as a contemporary psychiatric practice.

Its use is increasing. . . . It's more realistic today. Once a psychiatrist proved his worth by never using ECT. We're getting away from that overreaction. (geriatric psychiatrist)

ECT is neither barbaric, a punishment, nor insulting to patient or therapist. If used appropriately, it is a humane addition to a therapeutic program. (CSH ECT Manual)

In spite of its increasing use, and the specialists' confidence in its "appropriate" use, the empirical basis for its efficacy remains a complete mystery. Organic theorists postulate changes in the automatic nervous system and in the production of hormones. Psychoanalytic theories claim treatment in the form of fear and punishment, amnesia and relearning, and regression (Miller 1968; Cannicott 1968).

Depression and suicidal thoughts or acts are indicators for ECT. Because depression is considered to be a major psychiatric illness among geriatric patients (Feigenbaum 1974), ECT is particularly "appropriate" for the aged.

Furthermore, it is an attractive alternative to medication with deleterious side effects. "ECT is preferred to antidepressants because it doesn't have the dangerous side effects that so many meds have with the elderly" (psychiatric nurse, CHC).

The inpatient staff selects candidates for ECT who are then visited by the ECT consultation team. The team is composed of six first-year psychiatric residents, assigned for one month, and a permanent third-year resident. The patient is interviewed for 15 to 20 minutes. The residents ask leading questions about feelings of "hopelessness" and "helplessness." The patient's performance during the brief interview, the biased questioning, and the opinion of ECT novices are the basis for decision making.

ECT might be administered as often as three times a week to an inpatient (or intermittently to an outpatient). The patient, particularly one agitated about receiving ECT, may be sedated (given high doses of Librium or Valium, for example) early in the morning. Once the patient is escorted "downstairs," immediate preparations for ECT include anesthesizing and oxygenating the patient. A muscle relaxer is administered to reduced spinal compression, as severe compression will crack the patient's vertebral column.

There are three important variables in administering electrical current to the patient's brain: voltage, placement of electrodes, and duration of application. Voltage is potentially but infrequently modified by a glissando control knob on the electrostimulator, and marked in units, "low," "medium," and "high."* The electrostimulator itself is about the size of a toy train transformer. Two electrodes are placed either bilaterally or unilaterally. Bilateral, with electrodes placed above and in front of the ears, is the routine procedure. Unilateral, with one electrode placed at the center of the forehead, is for the less confused, less regressed patient. Proper location of the actual electrode placement is imprecisely defined. The duration of electrical stimulation varies from two to six seconds. Two residents are required to administer the electricity: one holds the electrodes and the other operates the electrostimulator. The operator switches on the current and then counts for a predetermined length: one-one thousand, two-one thousand, three-one thousand. Precision is not necessary.

The decision about duration and placement supposedly reflects the patient's ECT history and improvement. The team doctors, however, may be totally unfamiliar with the patients from the various hospital services. In at least one case, no one knew how the patient was progressing. Finally, one ward

---

*In the ECT I observed, the voltage was unchanged for four different patients, but in one candidate interview, an ECT team member recommended that they "go with low voltage" for a patient diagnosed as depressed but animated. Apparently modified voltage is an option, but it is infrequently used.

representative, a nurse, offered her estimation. On this basis, the patient received two seconds rather than three seconds of electrical current. The decision-making process is characterized by one ECT team first year resident: "We're like chefs—add a little garlic until it's just right" (psychiatric resident 7, CSH).

Finally, the grand mal seizure is considered to be an important part of the treatment. Improvement is supposedly related to length of seizure, but no one knows why. Length of seizure varies from five to sixty seconds. Because of the muscle relaxer, nearly imperceptible muscle twitching in the ankles and feet is the only evidence of it. The team doctors assiduously stare at the patient's feet. The first one to note the twitching announces, "There she goes," and the duration is recorded.

In approximately 20 to 30 minutes, the patient is sufficiently recovered to leave the room. Because of the emphasis on time-saving procedural efficiency, ECT team residents depart prior to the patient's recovery. They see neither the short-run nor long-run effects of their intervention. Ward staff escorts patients back to their ward as soon as possible. In one case a social worker needed my help in guiding an unstable walker down the hall. The sterile setting, emphasis on efficiency, and prompt retreat of residents maximize scientific impressions and minimize the practitioners' personal encounter with the patient.

Psychotherapy

The willingness of mental health professionals to engage elderly in psychotherapy depends on their belief in the rehabilitation potential of the aged in general. A portion of the geropsychiatric literature is highly optimistic about the fruitful application of psychotherapeutic techniques to the elderly:

> Older people are better able to postpone gratifications and are readier to acknowledge the inescapable contract: that one must perform in order to achieve. (Weinberg 1970)

> Elderly patients are highly responsive. The results are frequently more dramatic than with any other age group (Pfeiffer and Busse 1973).

Two therapeutic approaches are identified in the literature as having specific application to the aged, "supportive" and "reminiscence" techniques. Generally, supportive techniques demand a more active role on the part of the therapist (Pfeiffer and Busse 1973) and focus on resolving present problems and mastering present challenges rather than uncovering the past (Patterson 1971; Weinberg 1957). Noting a "predilection" for reminiscence in elderly, some practitioners (Butler 1963, 1973; Pincus 1970) have called for ". . .

psychotherapeutic intervention to enhance the life review process . . . to make it more conscious, deliberate, and efficient" (Butler 1974).

This perspective does not emerge at Central State Hospital because all elderly patients are diagnosed senile or organic brain disease. Psychotherapy cannot eliminate brain damage. Medication, ECT, and psychotherapy have a common trait: they are not curative of the senile condition. Of the three, only psychotherapy (or related themes) is not redefined as a stabilizing strategy, as its stabilizing potential is not seriously considered. The difference reflects the valuation of resources and their supply as much as the science of intervention.

Since one third of the Clairborne medical hospital beds are filled with elderly patients, it is not surprising that the elderly appear in large numbers at City Hospital. According to one medical resident: "We're pulverized, inundated with 82-year-old women" (medical resident 1, CH). Whether or not they are in need of medical care, many are confused.

> They bring all the confused old people here. (social worker 3, emergency room, CH)

> I would say about 25 percent of the elderly we see are demented. (medical resident 5, CH)

The appearance of confused elderly at the hospital door may provoke no formal action or, at an extreme, it may result in hospitalization and a "dementia workup": "You have to do a dementia workup to differentiate the treatable from nontreatable. That's the problem for a general medical hospital" (psychiatric nurse 5, CH). Some come to the hospital, not for medical care but to socialize. The main lobby, the visitors' waiting room, the emergency room, the outpatient clinics, and the coffee shops have regular elderly visitors, some of whom are confused.*

---

*I interviewed several elderly who sat in the hallways at City Hospital. It was not uncommon to encounter those whose speech was as confused or more confused than their senior counterparts in the nursing home and mental hospital.

There's one fellow who comes and sits outside our office every day. He's from a local nursing home. Everyone greets him, and he says hello. (social worker 4, CH)

She likes to sit in the medical clinic. She's established. (social worker 2, CH)

The hospital staff accepts them without complaint, and is proud of its tolerance. These elderly are regarded as fixtures in an informal social milieu that documents the hospital's benevolence.

Other elderly who are confused about their identity wander into the hospital or are brought in by police. The hospital runs an informal misplaced persons service.*

A lot come in who just don't know who they are, or where they are. (psychiatric social worker, CH)

An elderly man came to the clinic. He couldn't remember his name or address or phone number. We had him try to dial his own phone number. It took about an hour, but he finally did it. He lived with his sister, and we sent him home. She said he was perfectly O.K. when he got on the train that morning. (patient advocate, CH)

Some come to the hospital as conventional patients seeking outpatient medical care. The medical staff considers confusion to be incidental to the physical ailments under treatment. It only becomes a problem for them when it undermines their definition of sound medical practice. An elderly person is labeled confused if he or she indulges in medical indiscretions or inhibits the smooth performance of medical routines.

The senile are hard to work with. They answer the same question again and again. Sometimes they reach out and grab you. (medical resident 2, CH)

She's a confused elderly lady who's been in the hospital six or seven times with m.i.'s. Her problem is dietary indiscretion. She doesn't eat right, and then gets sick. (continuing care worker 2, PH)

As a result, the staff is sometimes forced to choose between denying a confused person the right to self-determination and failing to provide adequate medical care.

---

*Techniques for identifying misplaced confused elderly are look in their clothes, they usually have some name, either of a person or nursing home, listed on their clothes. Look inside the tongue of the shoe, the state hospital puts its stamp there. Call four or five nursing homes in the area where the person was found.

She wants to go home so badly. She could if we put a folli in. But she'd just tear it out. She needs supervision. (continuing care worker 2, PH)

A senile old man refuses to take eyedrops for his glaucoma. What should we do? If he doesn't take them, it'll get worse. (patient advocate, CH)

We want to do what we think is best for them. Say we have an old person who's a little confused, and we want him to go to a nursing home, but he wants to go home. So we place him in a nursing home, and he leaves, gets sick again, and comes back to the hospital. We're angry because he didn't keep our plan, but it wasn't what he wanted. (patient advocate, CH)

Some confused elderly arrive at the City Hospital emergency room as referrals from other community stations. These elderly may need medical attention, but they are more likely to be "management problems." The hospital staff defines these discharge referrals as "dumps" and the patients as "disposition problems." According to hospital staff, the dumps come primarily from nursing homes and occasionally from the more prestigious medical hospitals in the area.

We get the nursing home dumps, patients who have been disruptive. (psychiatric social worker, CH)

Once an old man arrived in a taxi, wearing a "johnny" and an overcoat. The johnny had a Claiborne General Hospital label on it. We called them, and they said they didn't know anything about him. They had no record of him. It was obviously a lie. (psychiatric nurse 3, emergency room, CH)

When you find an intravenous feeding site, you know they've come from another hospital. (nurse 1, medical ward, CH)

For these elderly and others who have no place to go, City Hospital operates a nursing home placement service. In fact, routing is the primary service offered to confused elderly by the medical hospital. "We're a clearinghouse for crazy old people with no place to go" (medical resident 1, CH).

THE PREVAILING POINT OF VIEW

Unlike the mental hospital, which is unified by a common psychiatric doctrine, the medical hospital is ideologically heterogeneous. Diverse and independent service stations, the medical specialties, for example, have individualized points of view regarding the confused elderly. The psychiatric is only one among many. Nonetheless, there is a general opinion about senility and dementia that has interdisciplinary credibility. First, physical and organic factors are emphasized and social and emotional elements are deemphasized.

The primary concern is the patient's physical well-being and his medical needs. Social and emotional needs are secondary. Old people with adjustment problems get little aid. They're just shipped out like a side of beef into some hole to die. (social worker 1, CH)

I think mental illness is all organic, if you could tie it up some way. (medical resident 1, CH)

Second, the medical profession advances a humanistic rhetoric:

Good health care for the aged recognizes the deeper human resources in life. (Harris 1975)

These persons can be helped immeasurably by elementary attention and medication, provided the attitude of the physician is one of genuine human interest. (Braceland 1974)

The results of a study by Spence (1968), however, indicated that medical students were more prejudiced against elderly than against any other minority group. This prejudice appears in physicians' unsympathetic characterizations of confused elderly.

We say there are two ways to identify these old people, with the "O" sign and the "Q" sign. If they lay there with their mouths open, that's the "O" sign. If their tongue hangs out because they've had a stroke, that's the "Q" sign. (medical resident 3, CH)

She's impossible to evaluate. She's a social menace. (medical resident 2, CH)

Third, the terms "senility" and "dementia" are general catchalls for confused, lethargic, withdrawn behavior.

Anyone who's disoriented and not expected to improve is called demented. (nurse 1, medical ward, CH)

People who are old and wornout are called senile. The aging process has caught up with them. (nurse 2, emergency room, CH)

An attitude of futility is the fourth element:

Staff just look at them and say they're unworkable. (social worker 2, CH)

Nobody can cure old age, not social intervention or whatever intervention. (psychiatric social worker, CH)

Nobody wants anyone who doesn't have potential. (nurse 3, medical ward, CH)

This point of view is not universally applicable throughout the hospital system. The exceptions, however, are a minority, and are not part of the mainstream of general medical practice. They are often expressed by non-professionals, such as students, patient advocates, and ambulance drivers. One organizational contingent of the hospital, the continuing care unit, also rejects and opposes the prevailing notions about dementia. (Its point of view will be developed in the last part of this chapter.)

Those who are opposed to dementia labeling exhibit less prejudicial attitudes toward elderly in general. Rather than presuming dementia, they give the elderly the benefit of the doubt.

We prejudge old people. We just assume they're confused. Most old people are not that senile if you spend a little time with them. If they can live out there on the street, they know what they're doing. (patient advocate, CH)

Half of them are senile because their bodies are dehydrated. They just need food and a place to live. Forget the psychiatric stuff. (ambulance driver, CH)

They provide alternative explanations for behavior others accept as symptomatic of dementia. Confused behavior is redefined as practical survival strategies. Personnel sometimes blame themselves or the hospital procedure for creating the appearance of confusion in the elderly.

We had an old lady in the clinic strapped onto a bed. She was screaming, insisting on talking to her nephew before entering the hospital. The staff said she was crazy, but the only reason it sounded crazy was because it interfered with our system. I wouldn't want to be admitted here without notifying my relatives. (student social worker, CH)

The initially docile patient may become troublesome with developing confidence. As he becomes more familiar with the setting, he's more willing to express his discomfort. (continuing care worker 1, CH)

Some old people either get lost or elope after a doctor assigns them to a clinic for a test, like blood, EKG, x-ray, etc. There was one old man who everyone thought was confused because he always eloped, but after he got to know me, he told me he was afraid of being on the street after dark, and that's why he left the hospital early. After I promised to take him home, we never had a problem with his eloping. (patient advocate, CH)

The prevailing and minority positions are fundamentally opposing points of view. Point of view is associated with role expectations and training. Personnel have an outlook that is compatible with the job they are expected to do. Job may be defined by organizational responsibilities or by the individual's (for example, the physician resident in training) personal agenda. Within the institution, contradictory decisions and staff conflict infrequently emerge. Those in the minority are also those with the least institutional authority. Lacking in power, those in the minority do not have a pervasive effect on the handling of confused elderly.

BACK DOOR TO THE HOSPITAL

The Setting

Approximately 25 staff persons plus consultants are in the emergency room at any one time. The floor nurses are young, energetic, and intensely proud of the quality of medical intervention they provide. Since the physicians and consultants are assigned to the emergency room on a rotation basis, the nursing staff knows best the workings of the service. Nurses are responsible for an efficient, smoothly functioning emergency room. Doctors who spend too much time in the nurses' station are prompted to get to work. Although nurses do not openly contradict attending physicians, they complain discreetly among themselves about physician callousness and lack of thoroughness. They are both the management and conscience of the emergency room.

As a treatment setting, the emergency room is unique. It is exempt from the principle of continuity of care. There are no resources to gather detailed community histories on arrivals. The staff does not consider this its responsibility. The elderly who are too confused to give a comprehensible explanation of their community situation are handled with inadequate information. In addition, patients may be treated, admitted, referred, or released without benefit of medical history because of an inefficient medical record system. Under such circumstances, reports from ambulance drivers and policemen are extremely important for purposes of identification, social assessment, and decision making. Furthermore, the emergency room is not obligated to follow up patients admitted, referred to a hospital service, or released directly from the floor. The emergency room is physically and organizationally isolated from the rest of the hospital. As a result, emergency room care is fragmented; medical and social history and follow-up alternatives are not taken into account.

Confused Elderly on the Floor

The patient waiting room in the emergency room is a place where confused elderly, alcoholics, and social deviants can loiter without harassment by authorities. A few of the elderly appear so frequently that the staff recognizes them on sight and has labeled them the "constants," "repeaters," or "routiners."

> We've had at least 24 episodes with her. State hospital won't admit her. They say she's not crazy. And she's not sick enough to be in a nursing home. She was at the Chronic Hospital, but they tied her to a chair because she lights fires. (psychiatric nurse 12, emergency room, CH)

Some arrivals claim to be in need of medical attention; others do not bother. Keeping warm, safe, and clean are problematic for confused elderly living on the street. They sometimes use the emergency room as a laundromat and temporary residence.

> Sonya comes to the emergency room to wash her clothes. One time when I walked into the ladies' room, she was standing there naked, washing her clothes in the sink. (nurse 3, emergency room, CH)

> We get an old Italian man in here every once in awhile on the weekends. His family just dumps him at our door. By Monday the family takes him home. (medical resident 3, CH)

The length of time anyone is allowed to "hang out" in the emergency room depends on his or her tenacity and ingenuity. Confused elderly are among the most successful. In the following example, an elderly lady managed to live in and around the emergency room for five days after being evicted from a public housing project.

> Louise arrived Friday afternoon, then left. The police brought her back Friday night. She'd been drinking, and had fallen. She was loud and belligerent, and refused to permit an examination. We didn't know what to do with her. She fought being checked out. She refused to go to a nursing home. The psychiatrist said she's senile but competent, so there was nothing we could do for her. By Saturday afternoon, she still hadn't mobilized herself so we admitted her. On Monday she was discharged, and ended up back here. Monday night we finally evicted her. We had a taxi cab take her to the Santa Maria, but she refused to get out of the cab so the driver brought her back here. She was here when I came to work this morning but she's gone now. (head nurse, emergency room, CH)

She left only when she wanted to, at the first of the month. Her Social Security check would have arrived at her mailing address and she no longer needed the emergency room for shelter.

All the emergency room staff resent and complain about such nonconventional and inappropriate use of an emergency room: "We want to run an emergency room, that is, a room where emergencies are handled. All the time you have in the back of your mind, 'What if a real emergency comes in?' " (psychiatric nurse, emergency room, PH). Nonetheless, their allegiance to a strictly professional definition of the situation is mitigated by their sympathy for the confused elderly.

> These people come to the emergency room because there's just no other place for them to go. (psychiatric nurse, emergency room, PH)

> They feel they're entitled to stay here. They don't have our middle-class perceptions about what a hospital is for. (psychiatric nurse 1, emergency room, CH)

Screening Confused Elderly

Routing, not treatment, is the primary function of the emergency room with regard to confused elderly. Because of the large numbers of elderly who enter and leave City Hospital (and Public Hospital), the decisions made in the emergency room have a significant aggregate effect on their routing in Claiborne as well as on the fate of many individuals labeled senile or demented.

A confused elderly person can enter the hospital as a medical problem or as a disposition problem. For the medical staff, this is the difference between an appropriate and an inappropriate admission: "The hospital is not supposed to do disposition admissions. It depends on the goodwill of the physician" (social worker 1, CH). The distinction, however, is artificial and manipulable, since the medical admission and the disposition admission are not mutually exclusive categories. Most confused elderly who arrive at the emergency room are likely disposition problems, and, according to the emergency room staff, examinations always reveal some chronic or acute physical impairment in need of medical attention. "According to her nephew, she didn't know where she was. He was afraid she'd set something on fire. We admitted her for her cardiac condition" (continuing care worker 2, PH).

Doctors must find medical justification for the admission in order to ensure the hospital's reimbursement. "Since Medicaid and Medicare won't pay for a disposition admission, the doctors usually do a workup to find some medical cause" (social worker 1, CH). When a continuing care worker wants to admit an elderly person for placement reasons, she lobbies with the medical staff: "We can usually find someone interested in running some tests. We can use that time to evaluate and find a placement" (continuing care worker 2, PH).

Even confused elderly applicants with a vested interest in the decision recognize the flexibility in the medical versus social definition of admission and attempt to manipulate it accordingly. For example, an elderly lady seeking shelter in the hospital asked the physician to consider her physical condition: "I have aneurism. You ought to let me in" (Louise). When she was refused admission, she considered the decision arbitrary and unfair: "That bastard. He could have let me in if he wanted to."

The physical condition of the prospective patient has been shown to be only one factor, and often an insignificant one, influencing admission to the hospital. Community residence may be more important. Since patients discharged from nursing homes must be replaced in another home, they are admitted. Furthermore, the emergency room staff believes that these confused elderly are discharged because they are management problems, not because they need emergency medical care. Nursing homes are accused of dumping these old people on the hospital and inventing symptoms to camouflage their real motives.

> When a management problem arrives from the nursing home, the referral sheet might read, "X has fallen out of bed. Is he injured?" or it might say, "High fever and change in level of consciousness." This is camouflage. When we call the home to say we're sending him back, they say, "Oh, we gave the bed away. We didn't expect him back." (nurse 4, emergency room, CH)

> We get a lot of nursing home patients on Friday afternoon. They like to get rid of their troublesome patients for the weekend. (psychiatric nurse 1, emergency room, CH)

> We got an old man with a note attached to him that said, "He is suicidal. Send him to the State Hospital." All he did was scratch his wrists with a fork. We thought it was exaggerated, but we admitted him as a disposition problem. We later learned from the weekend nurse in the home that it was a put-up job. (psychiatric nurse 1, emergency room, CH)

Even though suspicious of the nursing home referrals, the emergency room staff has no choice but to admit patients the home will not accept back. When the emergency room staff decides a nursing home's dumping is too blatant or too frequent, the admitting doctor will confront the home. "It's a real battle. The doctors don't want to admit the nursing home wanderers because there are no medical problems " (social worker 3, emergency room, CH). Exchanges between hospital and nursing home representatives can be acrimonious and antagonistic. The hospital staff's protests are usually futile, and result only in delaying the inevitable admission. If a referral arrives in the evening or on weekends, the delay can last for hours while the doctor tries to locate the nursing home administrator.

Nursing home personnel are convinced of the propriety of their actions and earnestly defend their decisions. From their point of view, the discharge to the emergency room is an exercise in caution, not deception. Furthermore, they accuse emergency room personnel of being insensitive and uncooperative.

> They're just beginners; they're just learning. They shouldn't challenge our judgments. We have many more years of experience. If we send someone to the hospital, it's because they need to be there. (house doctor, private physician 1)

> I have as little to do with City Hospital as possible. If we send a patient from the nursing home, they'll send him back. Sometimes we have to override their decision, and the patient may die a few hours later. (house doctor, private physician 1)

The hospital staff has public and private rationales for opposing admission. The primary problem, according to staff, is the shortage of beds. Metropolitan newspapers reported the major local hospitals are at least 95 percent filled. At City Hospital, the problem is particularly acute because of a recent reduction in the number of beds available.

> The number of beds has been drastically cut. We want to protect our open beds; save them for people who really need them. (medical resident 2, emergency room, CH)

> I wouldn't have any objections if he needed admission. I can appreciate the problems of the nursing home, but you can't believe what would happen if I sent him upstairs. There's one intern with 25 patients ready to die. It's worse here than in the nursing home, believe me. It's not fair to the patient or to the hospital. (medical resident 3, CH)

The problem at City Hospital is complicated by its open admission policy. In spite of a formal agreement among the hospitals to share the admissions, the staff complains about other hospitals' noncompliance and selective admission policies:

> There's a formal agreement but they don't always cooperate. Every other hospital can and does set admission standards. City Hospital serves a unique population, one which is hardly acceptable on the private hospital circuit. (social worker 1, CH)

The prohibitive cost of hospital care is another public rationale for opposition.

> We must do a physical examination on every admission—chest x-ray, clinical blood count, renal function, urinalysis, EKG—the whole thing! That's worth several hundred dollars. It probably costs $60 a day for a bed in the

hospital, so the total cost could come to between $300 and $800 for someone who doesn't really need medical care. (medical resident 3, CH)

The hospital is also viewed as a health hazard for the elderly.

Being in the hospital is a risk to the elderly's health. There's always the danger of infection. (psychiatrist, PH)

If he's admitted here, the chances of his leaving aren't good, unless it's to the morgue. (medical resident 3, CH)

In addition, there are private rationales taken for granted by insiders. City Hospital, like Public Hospital, is a teaching hospital. Any person admitted to the wards without complicated medical problems is a second-class patient: "This is a teaching hospital. The house staff wants something exciting. They don't want the run of the mill." (continuing care worker 1, PH). Confused elderly, who make little contribution to the on-the-job training of interns and residents, are undesirable from an educational point of view: "A confused elderly person is usually a disposition problem, and that's not very interesting for hospitals and doctors" (social worker 1, CH). Hospital policy requires basic medical diagnostic procedures that are time consuming, redundant, and uninteresting for the doctors: "Most interns don't want to admit senile because they don't want to do the workup" (medical resident 1, CH). All of the confused elderly are suspect. They may turn out to be both management and disposition problems on the medical ward and further burden an overextended staff.

For these reasons, admitting doctors are evasive and noncommittal when faced with an elderly admission. Ward assignment is negotiated among the staff physicians.

When an old person is likely to be a disposition problem, that patient will be seen by numerous consulting specialists. The medical consult will call the surgical, the surgical will call the orthopedic, they'll call the neurological, who will call the psychiatrist. There are two ways to understand this process. One, these specialists are trying to find the most appropriate ward for the patient. Two, everyone knows this patient will be a problem in treating and discharging, and no one wants the responsibility. (psychiatric nurse 2, emergency room, CH)

Maybe we can get her in upstairs if the admitting doc is asleep. (medical resident 5, CH)

If a confused person arrives directly from a private residence in the community, considerations underlying the admission decision are modified. The individual has the benefit of not being labeled a "dump," and is more likely to be viewed sympathetically.

These are old people who are weak and confused. They live in unsanitary conditions, have poor health, and are a hazard to their neighbors. (psychiatric nurse 2, emergency room, CH)

A senile old person will be admitted to the hospital even though there's nothing wrong with him. You can't send him out. He can't take care of himself. (psychiatric nurse 4, CH)

A confused elderly person might also be admitted for the purpose of observation without staff objection even though the need for medical attention is not apparent. Under circumstances of sympathy and uncertainty, the staff is predisposed to admit without exploring noninstitutional alternatives. In the following illustration, an elderly lady fell at home, cut her lip, was brought to the emergency room, and admitted solely for the purpose of observation, in spite of her protests and objections. The use of the Visiting Nurse Association to monitor her physical condition and evaluate her self-maintenance capability was suggested, but nothing was done.

Social worker 3: She needs to be admitted, and placed in a nursing home.
Medical intern 1: Why?
Social worker 3: She's 80.
Nurse 4: She's confused. She keeps repeating herself.
Social worker 3: She can't go home. She can't take care of herself.
Nurse 4: Can she walk?
[The lady was never given a chance to walk. Even that would have been a poor test since she used a walker at home and did not have access to one in the emergency room.]

Alternatives to Admission

Obviously not all the confused elderly who appear at the emergency room are admitted. A nursing home is sometimes willing, or is successfully pressured, to accept a returned patient. For confused elderly from private residences who are deemed unnecessary and undesirable admissions, the staff options are to stall, to displace, and to evict. There may be long delays in decision making. Some delays are unavoidable: "Sometimes it takes three or four hours just to get a blood report" (nurse 5, emergency room, CH). Other delays are manufactured by medical ward admitting doctors who hope to negotiate a reassignment of the patient while stalling.

It's no big deal for patients to wait four or five hours in the emergency room while services are bickering over who's going to take this one. (psychiatric nurse 2, PH)

The medical wards don't want them admitted, so they stall. They order all sorts of extra tests before they'll admit. (nurse 5, emergency room, CH)

Long delays may discourage the candidate, who eventually elopes.

No need to hurry to see her. We'll wait awhile, and if she doesn't elope, we'll tell her she's all right, and send her home. (nurse 3, emergency room, CH)

Nurse 1 (emergency room): Did she elope yet?
Nurse 2 (emergency room): I don't know. I gave her her clothes, and put down the bedrail.

The second option is to displace candidates. This occasionally involves referring them to another institution: "We were lucky in this case. The lady was crazy enough to send to the state hospital. Someone who was a little more put together would be a real problem" (psychiatrist 1, CH). More often, confused elderly are displaced by removing them to the waiting room:

It used to be we'd admit everyone, even the marginals. But because of the reduction in available beds, we're more conservative now. So rather than admit these people, they spend more time in the waiting room. (psychiatric nurse 1, emergency room, CH)

We put her in the waiting room. If she doesn't leave, the police will pick her up and dump her out on Center Street. She'll be around there until some other police find her wandering around, and bring her back to the emergency room. (nurse 2, emergency room, CH)

When confused elderly refuse to leave and the hospital refuses to admit, the staff forces eviction, as in the case of Louise, who stayed five days in or around the emergency room: "Medicine, surgery, the floor nurses, and social services have all agreed to evict her" (psychiatrist 2, CH). The psychiatrist has a special institutional role in the eviction of confused elderly: "They called me down for medical-legal reasons. The doctors decided to evict her, and they want me to document her competency as insurance against the risk of a complaint later" (psychiatrist 2, CH).

THE MEDICAL WARD

Confused elderly admissions usually go to the medical wards, not to psychiatry or neurology. The pattern is a consequence of hospital politics as well as medical judgment. "With confused old people, it's medicine versus neurology, and medicine always loses. That's the politics of the hospital" (psychiatric nurse, emergency room, PH).

A "dementia workup" is given on the medical ward, and the patient is labeled treatable or untreatable.

> If the elderly patient is confused, first locate the medical problems. It could be a diabetic condition that's causing the confusion. (nurse 1, PH)

> If it's organic, the doctors can screen it out right away. (social worker 3, CH)

> The purpose of the dementia workup is to rule out any treatable causes. (medical resident 1, CH)

A few of the treatable or semitreatable organic causes identified by medical ward doctors are dehydration, diabetes, electrolyte imbalance, tumor, certain diseases, elevated spinal fluid pressure, and dilated ventricles in the brain.

The dementia workup at City Hospital consists of the following examinations: blood test for venereal disease, vitamin B_{12}, toxic screens, and bromide level; spinal tap to look for disease (meningitis) and abnormal pressure; brain scan to pick up mass lesions and structural abnormality; and EEG to look for unusual functional activity in brain waves. Optional tests include pneumoencephalogram, a Roentgenographic picture of the brain after replacement of cerebrospinal fluid with air or gas to test for fluid blockages and dilated ventricles; resis scan, angiogram to map out the distribution within the brain of an intravenously administered radioisotope; and computerized axial tomography to measure brain atrophy.

Medical ward doctors do not perform their diagnostic tasks enthusiastically. As previously mentioned, they complain that the rest of the hospital has dumped the elderly on their ward. They also object to the hospital's "aggressive" dementia workup policy.

> They're very big on dementia workups here. Most interns don't like to do it, but if you don't, they get on you about it. (medical resident 1, CH)

> Whenever you get onset of confusion with a high fever, you must do a spinal tap. We've done a tap three times in the last three weeks on the same guy. (medical resident 5, CH)

The doctors are critical of the testing policy because there are unnecessary complications when a patient is "overworked"; both morbidity and mortality are associated with neurological testing; and with a less aggressive policy, diagnosis could be handled on an outpatient basis, thereby eliminating unnecessary admission. Furthermore, the doctors are critical because of their fundamental conviction that, regardless of test results, the confused elderly person suffers irreversible dementia and is therefore untreatable.

Usually we get a case where an old lady starts dumping on the floor, and the family brings her here. It's worthless to do a neuro workup on somebody like this. They're not reversible. (medical resident 1, CH)

No one has ever seen a dementia reversed, and still they keep pouring in here. (medical resident 1, CH)

Only one out of 300 resis scans are positive, and then the patient is generally untreatable because of being demented too long. (medical resident 1, CH)

Mental disorders are usually considered psychogenic when a workup fails to discover organic abnormalities (Wang 1973). With the elderly, however, either positive or negative results are accepted as evidence of dementia:

If no cause is found, they're diagnosed chronically stable dementia. (medical resident 4, CH)

When they do a workup, they seldom find anything, and they call it organic brain disease with hardening of the arteries. That's irreversible. (continuing care worker 2, PH)

In spite of popular thinking, the diagnosis does not prove senile dementia untreatable. At best, it fails to discover organic pathologies that can be treated under the domain of physical medicine. The breach in logic can be attributed to the prevailing physician attitudes cited above.

On the medical ward, the physicians have the institutional authority to make the definitive diagnosis of dementia. This is a statistical generality. The medical resident's diagnostic authority is superseded by the consulting psychiatrist. However, psychiatrists are rarely asked to consult on confused elderly unless the person is also a management problem. Still, according to them, an accurate diagnosis really depends on an adequate medical-social history: "Three quarters of any diagnosis is an adequate history" (medical resident 3, CH). In general medical practice, the level of intervention with acutely ill is based on the history of illness as well as the patient's present physical condition: "An elderly patient previously healthy but now acutely ill is more likely to be "four-plussed," that is, to receive intensive medical intervention, than is the chronic illness case with progressive decline" (physician 1, CH). When the same principle of intervention is applied to diagnosing dementia, acute onset, not diagnostic test results, is the deciding factor:

[A consulting psychiatrist had diagnosed an elderly lady organic brain syndrome, but the resident was skeptical about his accuracy.] She was admitted after an M.I. According to her daughter, she was never confused before she came to the hospital. Given the sudden onset and recent improvement in behavior, this seems like a very unlikely person to be termed "organic" in spite of the psychiatric diagnosis. Her only problems are a little wandering at night and a bad memory. (medical resident 1, CH)

Yet there is no reliable history for most confused elderly on the medical ward. Often the elderly patient does not give a coherent history. Other sources are considered inadequate or their accuracy is regarded with skepticism.

You get bad histories from families and nursing homes. That makes it difficult to distinguish between acute and chronic. (medical resident 5, CH)

Her husband *claims* [emphasis added] she was never like this before. (from the patient's medical record)

Doctors believe that confusion in the elderly is chronic and stable and that conflicting evidence is inadequate and unreliable. Therefore the confused elderly patient is without the means to challenge the institutional definition of dementia.

PSYCHIATRY: THE NONPARTICIPANT

As evidenced by the profusion of professional disciplines and diversity of services, the hospital takes seriously its claim to treat the whole person. According to popular medical opinion, the presence of a psychiatric service is essential to such holistic ambitions.

Psychological reactions to physical problems have the potential of interfering with treatment, and any attempt to not treat the whole patient but just the medical problem is doomed to unnecessary difficulties, if not failure. Psychotherapy should be a part of every comprehensive medical rehabilitation program. (Godbole and Verinis 1974)

A psychiatrist might find out something you didn't know. You just want to get as many resources as possible. (nurse 1, medical ward, CH)

Nonetheless, its role in servicing confused elderly is small.

In the manner similar to the psychiatric consultation in the nursing home, mental health specialists may be called on to contribute to diagnosing organic brain disease, senility, or dementia on the medical ward. The request is usually associated with management problems and the need for medication.

The issue of management is a large part of the psychiatric consultation. (social worker 1, PH)

The psychiatrists are useful for prescribing and making adjustments in medication. (continuing care worker 1, CH)

The psychiatric service is accused of being an elitist team that discriminates against undesirable patients, and the elderly and disruptive patients are
among the most undesirable.

We continually remind nurses to ask for psych consults, but they know the
psychs are only looking for the fascinating case. We're disillusioned with
their services. (continuing care worker 1, PH)

When I see a 75-year-old confused, senile person, I don't call the psych
department. They don't know how to deal with that type. (social worker 2,
CH)

As a result, the other hospital clinics are not only hesitant to call on psychiatrists but they are skeptical of the consultants' judgments.

We called for a psych evaluation. They said the patient isn't "actively
psychotic." That was no evaluation at all. They said he's competent because
he knows the date and who the President is. But how much does that have
to do with a patient being maintained in the community? (medical resident
5, CH)

The psych consult speculated it was organic, but you never know how much
of the "organic cause" is in the psychiatrist's mind. (medical resident 1, CH)

In response to these accusations, the staff at the psychiatric clinic asserts
that intervention would only duplicate the care of the ward staff:

The other clinics and hospital wards are staffed by competent people.
They're doing a great job of serving the emotional as well as physical needs
of their patients. Our services aren't needed for the uncomplicated cases.
(psychiatrist 1, CH)

Furthermore, they take the same futilistic point of view as their counterparts
in the mental hospital: "Nothing can cure old age, not social intervention or
whatever intervention" (psychiatric social worker, CH). The psychiatric specialists also complain that the frequent requests for placement assistance are
inappropriate:

We aren't specialists at disposition. Other services can do it as well as we
can, in fact, better. If a nursing home gets a call from the psych clinic, it's
a strike against you. If the call is made from a primary care clinic, then the
patient is OK. (psychiatric social worker, CH)

PLACEMENT ORGANIZATION

The continuing care unit, consisting of six public health nurses and a social worker, is the principal component in the placement organization. Ward social workers and, to a lesser extent, ward doctors also have an important part. Only the continuing care staff claims to have regular face-to-face contact with the nursing home. One fifth of their time is spent in the community. They have authority to follow up discharged elderly and to investigate the adequacy of nursing home care. Corresponding to their unique role, they have a point of view concerning the confused elderly that contradicts the prevailing orientation. They take issue with such widely accepted tenets as:

Senility is irreversible

Very sudden and dramatic changes do occur in an older person's mental status. (continuing care worker 1, CH)

She looked like a classic senile confused case. With feeding and supervision, she came out of it. Now she's trying to make the decision about nursing home placement herself. (continuing care worker 2, PH)

You can reorient anyone by talking to him a few minutes each day. (continuing care worker 1, CH)

Organic changes in the brain cause senility

If an old person is confined to bed, all he or she sees is the white sterile environment, white walls, nurses in white. The result is confusion and disorientation. (continuing care worker 1, CH)

We add to their confusion. We isolate them, and shift them from place to place on stretchers so they don't know where they are. (continuing care worker 2, PH)

At times the continuing care staff even incorporated the patient's definition of the situation into their own point of view. For example, an elderly man on the orthopedic ward who was identified as senile wanted to lie down, but no one would help him. An attendant said she would be back in five minutes. No one explained to him that they wanted him to sit up in order to "clear his lungs." The continuing care worker observed: "That may be the worst of all —the frustration of having no one pay any attention to you. You're not really out of it and not completely together, but well enough to know that no one's listening" (continuing care worker 1, CH). Only the continuing care unit found the professional response to the confused elderly deplorable and objected to even the social uses of the term "senility": "Senility. I don't like the word, and I don't want the nurses in this unit to even use it" (continuing care worker 2, CH).

The ward social workers' role is limited to handling bureaucratic procedures. They do not initiate any social treatments for hospitalized elderly; nor
do they participate in any, since none exist. They do not go into nursing homes
to follow up discharged patients. Their job is to explore a patient's financial
resources and arrange, when appropriate, for public financing of aftercare.

> We look for resources—Medicaid, SSI, pension savings, private income, and
> so on. (social worker 1, CH)

> We initiate the Medicaid application through Welfare. (social worker 1, CH)

At City Hospital, the social worker is also responsible for making the final
selection of the nursing home from a list of recommended homes submitted
by the continuing care workers.* The social workers understand their contribution in the selection process to be a respect for the social dimension otherwise neglected.

> Nurses in continuing care generally focus on the medical needs of the patient
> and their knowledge of the medical skills of the various homes when they
> make a recommendation. In making our choice we also consider the social
> factors. (social worker 1, CH)

The actual preparation for discharge involves the patient's doctor, the
ward social worker, and the continuing care nurse. Ideally, preparation begins
at admission. "Cardex rounds" and case conferences were initiated to keep the
placement organization up to date on a patient's arrival and progress. Decision
making is encumbered by the precarious relationships among the various
professionals. Officially, doctors make the discharge decision and aftercare
plan. They have both authority and superior status. In practice, they rely
heavily on the social workers to determine appropriate Visiting Nurse Association or home health care follow-up. In one case, the social worker merely
handed the attending physician a completed application for home health care,
which he signed and then asked: "What does a home health worker do anyway?" (medical resident 5, CH).
   The placement organization also complains that doctors are not interested
in aftercare and are deliberately negligent in filling out transfer and referral

---

*At Public Hospital, the continuing care unit is responsible for contacting the nursing homes.
This arrangement is more in keeping with the structure of interorganizational associations. It also
follows the patient's medical status in the hospital more closely. The explanation given at City
Hospital for the organization of tasks is that the continuing care unit is just too busy to contact
homes.

forms. The house doctors resent questioning of their competence and authority, and the result is mutual animosity:

> There's nothing worse than a social worker who tries to tell you your job.
> (medical resident 5, CH)

> This morning one of the house doctors referred to me as "that bitch of a
> social worker." I was after him to complete the nursing home transfer form.
> (continuing care worker 1, PH)

Timing is critical for the placement organization. Homes will not hold
beds for two or three days unless the patient is someone they know and want.
Social workers cannot call homes until the day of discharge or one day before.
It may also take several days to prepare a Medicaid application. Thus, physician cooperation is essential to social workers. "If they don't tell you until the
last minute, then you're in trouble" (social worker 1, CH). When patients are
medically stable, the ward doctors want them out immediately, especially if
every bed is filled and new patients must be "boarded out."

The utilization review committee is responsible for policing unnecessary
stays in the hospital. Its influence can be either evaded or manipulated by
practitioners according to their needs. In spite of its officially designated
authority, the committee's independent regulatory power is questionable.

> The family is reluctant to pay for nursing home care. But they don't want
> to take her home. We've already kept her for a long time. Now we'll put
> more pressure on them by having the utilization review committee terminate
> her stay. We might ask the family to take her home until she's placed. (social
> worker, Community Hospital)

> Some old people stay for weeks while we try to find a place. The utilization
> review committee says, "You must move this patient out," and the doctors
> try to fudge as much as they can. They say more diagnostic tests are needed,
> and they blame the continuing care nurses for not finding a placement
> sooner. (psychiatric nurse, emergency room, PH)

Utilization review committee pressure to discharge, however, might also be
requested by hospital staff when a family refuses to cooperate with discharge
plans.

> Sometimes you get extended hospital stays while the family works through
> ambivalence of what to do. Then a miniconfrontation may be necessary. We
> say, "The utilization review committee insists on discharge. You must do
> something." (psychiatrist, PH)

A Problematic Specialty

The placement organization's role as a specialist in the medical hospital relies on the existence of substantial dissimilarities among nursing homes. The worker must be able to recognize these differences and place patients accordingly. The first level of discrimination differentiates "good" homes from "bad" homes, and preference is given to the good homes. Some homes are unofficially blacklisted and never used. A second discriminating category considers "nursing" care and "social or recreational" care in the home. Quality is not necessarily uniform on these variables within the home.

> Some homes give excellent nursing care but zero social, recreational care. Or it's exactly the opposite. (continuing care worker 3, PH)

> The Autumn is a good home for physical care, but not very good for people's heads. Their people eat well and are ambulated regularly, but they make no decisions for themselves. (continuing care worker 2, PH)

Discriminate selection also takes into account idiosyncratic tolerances for specific kinds of deviant behavior. A home might be judged unwilling or unable to deal with one or more of the following: incontinent patients, drinking problem patients, disruptive patients, patients with colostomies, wandering patients, or "psychiatric" patients.

Ideally, placement matches home characteristics and preferences with the patient's medical, social, and personal characteristics. For example, patients with more complicated medical problems would go to the nursing homes with higher quality nursing care. Placement should also consider geographic proximity to the family and/or neighbors because "Friends, family, and neighbors will visit only if it causes a minimum inconvenience" (social worker 1, CH). The availability of crafts, activities, and recreation should be matched with the patient's need for involvement and activity.

> Is the patient a loner or does he want to play beano? (continuing care worker 3, CH)

> How much attention does the patient want? Does he want someone to tell him what to do or recognition of independence? (continuing care worker 3, CH)

The placement organization is cognizant of the impact that home selection may have for the patient, and is seriously committed to making the "best" placement possible: "When there's no family, the onus is on the social worker to make the very best placement possible. Your decision may influence where the patient will spend the next five or ten years of his life" (social worker 1, CH).

The idealized concept of the placement selection is, however, difficult, if not impossible, to put into practice. To reiterate, timing the patient's recovery rate, the hospital discharge, and the nursing home's acceptance is precarious under the best of circumstances. Sudden changes in the patient's mental or physical status may disrupt all discharge plans: "We had him all set to go when he got a case of the 'no eats.' Now we have to start over" (social worker 1, CH). Doctors, social workers, and continuing care workers all have complaints about each other's performance of discharge obligations. A smooth, co-operative, teamlike functioning has not yet been realized. At worst, desperation replaces cooperation: "We do battles with doctors not to discharge until suitable placement arrangements have been made. Sometimes they discharge patients on Saturday when we aren't here" (continuing care worker 1, PH).

There are over 30 nursing homes in Claiborne and hundreds in the metropolitan area that the continuing care unit can recommend. Quality of care in nursing homes is unstable, fluctuating primarily with changes in nursing home personnel. With a staff of six, the continuing care unit cannot keep up to date or supply detailed information on the quality of care in all those homes. A confused elderly person may need extensive supervision, which the majority of Medicaid homes does not provide.

> Usually organic brain syndrome patients require total care. However, they have few skilled nursing needs. So they can't go to a Medicare-financed skilled nursing home, but the non-Medicare homes, the level three's, don't have the staff to provide total care. So how do you place them? (continuing care worker 1, PH)

The "matching" concept does not fully recognize the discriminatory power of the nursing home. Every home takes into account what the continuing care workers call the "big three" variables: is the patient continent, a self-feeder, and ambulatory? Some confused elderly, such as the wanderers and screamers, are extremely difficult to place in any home: "Her problem is nobody wants a screamer. The previous social worker tried three different times to place her" (continuing care worker 2, CH). Nursing homes have the opportunity to select since the demand for beds greatly exceeds the existing supply.

> I called 25 homes before I found one. (social worker, Community Hospital)

> If a home has empty beds, it's because no one wants to send patients there. (continuing care worker 1, PH)

As a result, the placement organization's opportunity to select the most desirable home, once it is specified, is very small. It is as accurate to say that the home chooses its patients as that the hospital's placement organization selects the home. For the placement organization, it is mostly a matter of taking what it can get .

V

SOCIAL POLICY

Twenty years ago older people diagnosed as senile dementia or organic brain syndrome shared a common fate. These elderly, whether they arrived in their youth or were admitted in their later years, would spend their remaining days confined to the back wards of state mental hospitals. Their life space was restricted to a dayroom and a dormitory in a total institution that was physically and socially isolated from mainstream society. Among other benefits, the movement toward community care promised alternatives for those who would have been hospitalized. It promised ex-institutionalized patients the opportunity for relearning social roles through more diversified and complex community associations. In return for this new life space, patients would suffer temporary relocation discomfort, but that would be minimized by professional discharge planning.

For confused elderly, the goal of new community associations has been achieved, even if unintentionally, by routing them perpetually from station to station. In exchange for the back ward, a confused elderly patient may experience numerous nursing home placements and short-term stays in a medical or mental hospital.

We had one guy who had just worn out the nursing home circuit. (psychiatric social worker, CH)

I have one lady who has been in six different homes in the last two years. She's discharged from the hospital to the home, she cuts up after a few months, and is returned to the hospital. She prefers the hospital, and she likes to come back. (welfare worker 3)

There are the "routiners" who escape from their nursing homes, and end up here. Sooner or later they exhaust their supply of nursing homes. (nurse 2, emergency room, CH)

Claiborne social agents' metaphorical characterizations leave no doubt that they think the institutional referral system is inadequate.

Old people are just moved around like so much rotten fruit. (administrator, Thompson Nursing Home Corporation)

It's just like dropping a hot potato. Maybe someone will stop and pick it up. (psychiatric nurse, emergency room, PH)

They ship them out of here as if they were a side of beef. (social worker 1, CH)

The terminology most frequently used describes the discharge and referral process as a "dump job." While no station admits to dumping, they all claim to be dumped on.

Friday afternoon is dump day. Sometimes it seems like we have a representative from every home in the area. (psychiatric nurse, emergency room, PH)

When a nursing home is looking to get rid of a patient, they know where to do it. (psychiatric nurse 9, CSH)

The emergency room staff is always accusing Central State of dumping their patients over here. (continuing care worker 1, PH)

City Hospital sends all their disposition problems over here. (psychiatric nurse 10, CSH)

Confused elderly in transit are also described as being "bounced around." Even if they are referred to another station, they may be bounced back: "Many of the old people we send over to Central State aren't admitted. I don't know what they offer as an alternative. Sometimes they just bounce back over here" (psychiatric nurse, emergency room, PH).

As can be seen in Figure 1, every station is faced with numerous referral and discharge options. What is perceived by station managers and labeled as bouncing or dumping is the continual cyclical movement of Claiborne confused elderly through the community stations. This, community movement has created, in effect, a loop, capable of routing the person perpetually until he or she lands temporarily in some institutional niche, leaves the community, or dies.

Movement on the loop can be initiated or furthered by any of the participating agents.

Central State Hospital tried to place a patient several times. Each time he came back. He's really demented. He's also been treated at Public Hospital for acute illness. He was finally placed in a home we don't use. He was

FIGURE 1

Flowchart of the Processing System for Confused Elderly

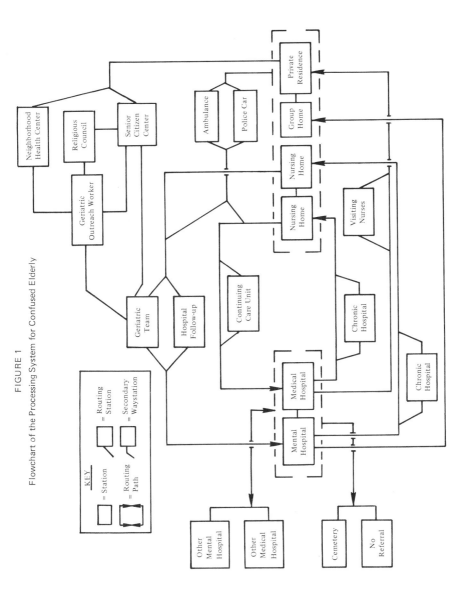

"posied" there, and he became bedridden. His skin broke down, and he came here. Public Hospital refused to take him. Central State wouldn't take him because he's nonambulatory. So we'll treat him and place him. (social worker 1, CH)

The deinstitutionalization of state mental hospitals introduced many confused elderly to the community loop rather than to stable community residences. The hospital emergency room receives confused elderly from nursing homes who are acutely ill or injured or who have been discharged under the pretext of a medical emergency. The medical hospital is an acute care setting, and only short-term stays are permitted to "stabilize" elderly. Unless a patient has an excellent conduct record in the home and a very brief stay in the hospital, the nursing home will fill the vacated bed before the ex-resident can be returned. Usually the patient must be relocated in another home. The mental hospital is no longer a chronic care institution. If admitted, the elderly patient's stay there is also temporary. Old people who appear at the mental hospital door are more likely to be routed than admitted. Families, landlords, and neighbors evict confused elderly who have become too troublesome to handle at home.

> I heard her screaming and yelling upstairs. She lived on the top floor, and complained about the people who lived above. She'd use language that even a sailor wouldn't use. There were so many complaints, they had to get rid of her. (senior citizen 8)

> We get calls from landlords to evict old people. We tell them if the person's competent, we aren't going to violate their civil rights. If they know who and where they are, they're competent. (ambulance driver, CH)

No confused elderly person is free from the threat of being put on the loop. Even nursing home "pets" fall from their favored positions if their behavior becomes chronically troublesome. There are no institutions offering end-of-the-line services as part of their stated function. The medical hospital indirectly serves this purpose when the seriously ill are sent to the hospital to die. Also, the mental hospital has made exceptions in its short-term care doctrine for a very few: "No one else will keep her. We've decided to let Margie stay here until she dies" (chief resident, Service A, CSH).

The two chronic hospitals serving Claiborne and the metropolitan area will accept the end-of-the-line role if a patient's life expectancy is short, if a patient has been continually looped until the supply of nursing homes is exhausted, or if a patient's behavior is so bad that nursing home placement is impossible: "She's been in and out of six different nursing homes. Now she's going to the Chronic Hospital. She'll stay there until she dies. Even she said, "Well, I guess it's the end of the line for me" (welfare worker 3). The chronic hospitals also screen their patients for discharge and make placements in nursing homes, so they also contribute to looping.

Once a confused elderly person is on the loop, there are few escapes. Institutional organizations do not discharge them back to their homes. "Since I've been here, I've seen only one old person go home after hospitalization, and she had lots of community contacts" (social worker 2, CSH). Many professionals responsible for placement clearly have a bias favoring institutional placement. Going home is assumed to be an inferior service alternative.

> You know, when you see them you wonder how they ever managed to survive outside. You feel you can't send them back. So what are you saying to them, "Let us offer you our clean white sheets in exchange for your freedom and privacy." (continuing care worker 2, PH)

> Should a person be placed in a nursing home or struggle to stay in an apartment? In a nursing home a patient can use energies previously devoted to self-maintenance for leisure and recreation. (psychiatrist, PH)

> The moment anything goes wrong, the tendency is to place them. (community worker, NHC)

ROUTING DILEMMA

With so many agencies and institutions participating in screening, handling, and referring confused elderly, it is important to address the question of which confused elderly go where and for what reason. The effect of station ideology and self-defined function on routing confused elderly has been discussed in Chapters 3 through 9. This chapter examines organizational "behavior" as it affects placement decisions.

A Clinical Perspective

The clinical perspective provides one explanation of routing phenomenon.* Clinicians assume that characteristics of the patient are the deciding factors in routing. The patient has a real problem, defined as a pathology, which the clinician diagnoses or evaluates. Furthermore, it is assumed that the different approaches taken by stations on the loop are a response to an obvious

---

*I am not suggesting that all clinicians, in all settings, share this point of view. Important differences have been elaborated in the preceding chapters. My purpose here is to generalize about the clinician's prevailing interpretation of the routing process.

differentiation in clients' characteristics and needs. On the basis of these needs, clinicians, particularly placement specialists, can intervene or direct individuals to the most appropriate station (Greenley and Kirk 1973; Gaitz 1974). Patient cooperation and satisfaction is taken for granted:

> We assume that the needy person recognizes his need and is quite ready to accept a service if and when it is provided, implying thereby that the need for the service is known, that it is possible to provide it, and that a provider is available. That the service will benefit the recipient and that other persons, significantly related to him, agree with, understand, and will cooperate in whatever ways are advantageous or beneficial to the needy individual is accepted without question or reservation. (Gaitz 1974)

When clinicians are confronted with continual discrepancies between their conception of routing and the widespread recognition that confused elderly are dumped and bounced around, they have their own qualifying and absolving explanations. These range from the old-fashioned "muddling through" optimism to the esoteric analysis of "systems."

> It may seem disorganized, but old people get where they belong. (psychiatric nurse 1, emergency room, CH)

> Professionals don't always agree on diagnosis or the best possible disposition. All we can do is follow our professional standards. (psychiatrist, PH)

> Patients deliberately set institutions against each other. They present contradictory symptoms which lead to conflicting diagnoses. (psychiatrist, PH)

The clinical concept, even with disclaimers, does not explain why the loop exists or why practitioners claim their community colleagues are engaged in widespread dumping. The uncertainty of diagnosis must be examined as one causative factor in the breakdown of the clinical perspective. Most applicants for social services, particularly the elderly, have multiple problems that can be classified in any number of ways. Applicants themselves are unsure of the nature of their problems and offer little guidance. As a result, clinicians have a wide latitude in defining the "real" problem (Kirk and Greenley 1974). More to the point, the data indicate that diagnostic procedures do not differentiate irreversible dementia from a temporary confused state, a distinction crucial to routing decisions. At best, the procedure can produce ex post facto judgments: if senile symptoms vanish, the old person was not demented. Under such circumstances, communitywide agreement about a single agency's screening and routing decisions is not achievable. The definition of the patient's problem and the appropriate response must be based on more than ambiguous clinical judgments.

An Organization Perspective

An alternative explanation of routing phenomenon can be constructed by examining the confused elderly's movement through the entire loop. This approach has a holistic advantage over the clinician's perception, which is limited to observing the arrival and departure of confused elderly from one setting. From a holistic perspective, principal routing determinants are the characteristics of organizations rather than the characteristics of the patient's pathology.

The managers of Claiborne stations involved in routing confused elderly have defined their organizations' functions in a manner that excluded handling most of them. These rationales explain why admitting (or treating or keeping) an undesirable elderly person would be misguided, inappropriate, or even irresponsible. Excerpted below are exclusionary rationales offered by some agents:*

Senior citizen centers

> I sympathize with the seniors. This is the main meal of the day for them. They can't sit next to someone who smells and eats food from others' plates. (senior citizen center director 1)

Families

> Families bring in old people who are bizarre, and want them committed. (psychiatric nurse 1, emergency room, CH)

> If there's a family, they're usually upset, and want to get rid of the person involved. (social worker 1, CH)

Nursing homes

> We can't take too many of the state hospital patients. They're disruptive, and we want to make things as homey as possible. (head nurse, Holst Nursing Home)

> Mixing the mental weakness patients with the better functioning is the primary problem in the nursing home today. (private physician 3)

---

*There were only two exceptions to the general use of defined function to reject confused elderly. One was the nursing home organizer, but that group played no part in the routing of Claiborne confused elderly. The Geriatric Specialist Team was the other. It did not so much exclude confused elderly as work around them. The influence of its peacekeeping operations on the movement of confused elderly was discussed in Chapter 5.

Police

If you're in the city, you're going all the time. Say you get a call for a suffocating infant while you're acting as a taxi for a lost old lady. Then you have a problem. (policeman 1)

Central State Hospital

The senile *officially* belong in nursing homes. (psychiatric resident 1, CSH)

What could you do for that kind of person? How could you give her psychotherapy? All the psychotherapy in the world wouldn't help her. (psychiatric nurse 5, CSH)

The medical hospital

Being in the hospital is a risk to the elderly's health. There's always the danger of infection. (psychiatrist, PH)

The old people come to the emergency room because there's no other place to go, but we want to run an emergency room, that is, a room where emergencies are handled. All the time you have in the back of your mind, "What if a real emergency comes in?" (psychiatric nurse, emergency room, PH)

Without the organizational means for discretion in admission, rationales would be useless in detouring undesirable arrivals. This discretion is sometimes referred to as boundary control (Greenley and Kirk, 1973). Evidence that all social agencies exercise boundary control is presented by Stuart Kirk and James Greenley. (1974). They observed that the percentage of applicants rejected ranged from 10 to 65 percent, and concluded that the variation was attributable to the organization itself rather than to its clients.

Boundary control was a readily apparent property of stations in Claiborne. At City Hospital there was a great deal of staff complaint about the minimal use of barriers at points of admission, particularly in the emergency room. The official open-door policy created overpopulated medical wards, and necessitated employment of a sophisticated continuing care unit and placement organization. City Hospital processed more confused elderly than any other station in spite of intensive internal complaint. Yet, the most transparent illustration of boundary control in action came from this station. Under the new stricter commitment law in this state, a person can only be committed who is suicidal, homicidal, or so disorganized he cannot take care of himself. In the following unusual case, however, all three conditions were fulfilled, and still the applicant was rejected.

An elderly lady arrived in the ambulance with her dead adult daughter. The ambulance driver said the daughter had been dead for several days. The mother's mumbling about "sheets" and "suffocating" led nurses to speculate about a possible homicide. [The daughter was an invalid requiring total bed care.] The mother talked about hearing noises inside her head and stomach. She also talked about suicide, saying, "I'm going home and drink myself to death." The psychiatric nurses concluded that she was "getting psychotic." However, the consulting psychiatrist refused to admit her because, "We have no medical reason for admission." The lady was discharged to an alcoholic son in spite of his objections. No mention was made of follow-up responsibility. Social worker 3 concluded, "The whole thing is crazy." (observer)

The dump, a manipulated displacement strategy, is evidence of exit boundary control. Staff's complaints about other stations' selective admission policies illustrate entrance boundary control.

Central State never wants to accept anyone, anytime. (psychiatrist 1, CH)

Central State won't ever take a confused elderly person. (continuing care worker 1, PH)

Nursing homes aren't supposed to discriminate, but they do. (social worker 1, CH)

Allowing for variations in degree of effectiveness, boundary control is a commonplace organizational trait. Ability, incentive, and rationale make possible widespread discrimination against confused elderly. Stations with weak boundary control are at a disadvantage in negotiating routing decisions with other stations on the loop. City Hospital is as unbounded as any station serving Claiborne. Patients arrive in taxi cabs from more exclusive medical hospitals. City Hospital cannot force nursing homes to take back a patient sent to the emergency room. Once a rejected patient is on its premises, it cannot displace the patient to another station at its own choosing. It is pushed into "medically inappropriate" admissions of rejects from other stations. As a result, the hospital is effectively servicing other stations rather than individual patients. Police have a similar problem when landlords insist that confused elderly tenants be removed. The police must respond to persistent neighborhood pressure, yet they cannot confidently transport deviants to a treatment station and be assured of their admission.

MANAGING THE REFERRAL IMPRESSION

Each station struggles to preserve its "appropriate function" by limiting access of confused elderly. The sum effect of individual (organizational) evasion is to create multiple referrals and repeaters, thereby enlarging the total number of referrals. Each station contributes to the loop the same effect that it wants to avoid for itself. As a loop participant, the station indirectly suffers the consequences of its own discrimination. The problem is self-perpetuating and beyond resolution through self-adjustment.

> We've held conferences to negotiate the handling of patients between our institutions. But it's hard to work out general guidelines we can follow. The best we can do is let each other know, case by case, what position we will take. (continuing care worker 2, PH)

Stations do not recognize the legitimacy of each other's exclusionary rationales, and will attempt the referral in spite of receiving stations' objections: "You'd think the state hospital would appreciate what we do for them, rather than only grudgingly accept patients that rightfully belong to them" (psychiatrist 1, CH). As a result, the exchange of patients among stations is accompanied by mutual hostility and aggressive boundary control. The acrimonious exchange between doctors in the City Hospital emergency room and the nursing home administrators (see Chapter 9) is one example. In a similar tone, a physician at City Hospital analyzed a state hospital referral: "Central State doesn't give a truck load of shit about the older patient" (medical resident 2, CH). Stations accuse one another of using tricks and gimmicks to detour confused elderly, and describe in militant terms the interorganizational associations:

> We still have battles with nursing homes. (psychiatric resident 1, CSH)

> Our relationships can turn into warfare when we treat from behind our own battlements. (psychiatric resident 3, CSH)

Under these circumstances, the station originating a displacement does not have the benefit of the receiving station's confidence. In order to minimize opposition and possible refusal, the originator promotes the legitimacy of the displacement decision by using impression management techniques. It is advantageous for the station to give the impression of trying to make an appropriate referral so that the receiving station will voluntarily act in accordance with its plans. When an institution discharges a patient, it is important that the person's appearance lead others to believe he has received competent and considerate care. If not, the institution's credibility is besmirched. It is particularly important for nursing homes, since their quality of care is generally suspect. But even this impression is not above suspicion. The arrival of a well-kept nursing home discharge in the hospital emergency room led an admitting doctor to comment: "The nursing home is careful to spruce up a patient before they send him out. They'll go over his face with an electric razor, bathe him, put on a clean johnny, and an ID bracelet" (medical resident 3, CH). When the movement of confused elderly is in the opposite direction, nursing homes accuse the hospital of "misrepresenting" patients. They suspect the placement organization conceals facts in order to make the patient appear to be "better" than he is.

> I got a false report. The state hospital didn't give the full truth. They just want to get the patient out of their bed. (head nurse, Holst Nursing Home)

> When I got a call from City Hospital I knew who they wanted to place, so I said, "I know you're calling about Mr. Smith, but you weren't going to tell me what a problem he is, that his family can't handle him, that he makes a lot of noise, and is intolerable." (head nurse, Holst Nursing Home)

In order to give an impression of integrity in spite of accusations of concealment, the placement organization explains discrepancies between its patient description and the nursing homes' perceptions.

> We must visit a patient as close as possible to the time of discharge because sudden and dramatic changes do occur. If our description of the patient is inaccurate, the nursing home complains that we misrepresented the patient. I always make them out to be a little worse than they are, then I'm safe. (continuing care worker 1, CH)

Hospital staff also accuses nursing homes of misrepresenting patients so that confused elderly will appear to be eligible for admission to a medical hospital:

> The home sent him in on Friday night, saying he wouldn't eat. Saturday morning he has an excellent appetite. (nurse 1, medical ward, CH)

> Nursing homes like to get rid of their troublesome patients. . . . They send them in with some medical excuse like high fever. (psychiatric nurse 1, emergency room, CH)

The exchange of impressions and challenges to impressions becomes so complicated that the supposed relationship between the clinician's assessment of pathology and the referral decision is completely obscured.

Labeling is fundamental to managing the referral impression. For the medical hospital, a successfully applied label accomplishes a rationalization for removal of the confused elderly individual: "It works like this. If you can't get a coherent conversation out of them, then they're senile. If they're senile, it doesn't matter where they go" (medical intern, CH). The dementia label is generally a sanction for nursing home placement: "He's senile. He should be in a nursing home" (psychiatric nurse 3, emergency room, CH)

Sometimes the label is used to advance a referral to the mental hospital:

> The psychiatrist admitted an elderly lady who had fallen down her stairs. He diagnosed her senile, and tried to get her admitted to the state hospital. She wasn't though. She's on the medical ward now, and doing just fine. (psychiatric nurse 3, emergency room, CH)

Central State Hospital staff also recognizes the importance of labels and their manipulation in determining the movement of confused elderly: "The senile officially belong in nursing homes. They're called 'organic brain syndrome,' a psychiatric diagnosis, and sent to the mental hospital. But they don't belong there" (psychiatric resident 1, CSH). As in the medical hospital, labels are manipulated to displace confused elderly. Organic brain damage is not considered a mental health problem: "Old people with chronic brain syndrome are just out of it. They don't need to be in a mental hospital. It probably wouldn't do them any good anyway" (psychiatric nurse 6, CSH).

The use of tranquilizers with disorderly elderly also contributes to the referral impression and routing process. Medical and mental hospital placement organizations are able to discharge some confused elderly otherwise "unpresentable" to nursing home admitting officers: ". . . she became a management problem, and we treated her with low doses of Haldol, and sent her to a nursing home" (psychiatric nurse 1, CSH). When homes and hospitals disagree on proper dosage, medication contributes to the routing problem rather than resolves it.

> When an old person is in the mental hospital, he gets massive doses of tranquilizers. The sedated patient returns to the nursing home. The house doctors don't use heavy doses so they write reduced medication orders. The patient acts up, and is returned to the hospital where his medication is once again increased. The cycle begins again. (welfare worker 3)

Tranquilizers are used inside nursing homes not to accomplish a referral, but to avoid a discharge. The purpose of the medical adjustment is to help disorderly residents give a new impression that they are the kind of cooperative patients the staff wants to keep: "Will medication control? That's the only question. If the patient can be managed with medication, then everything is all right. (private physician 1, house doctor, Court Nursing Home).

To summarize, the distinction between a dump and a referral is indicative of no more than contrasting points of view. Managing the impression of a referral necessitates the use of communication strategies—concealment, labeling, tranquilizing—through which social agents seek to impose their own definitions of the situation on others. The issue is not defining the appropriate referral, but establishing what Goffman calls a "working consensus":

Together the participants contribute to a single overall definition of the situation which involves not so much a real agreement as to what exists, but a real agreement as to whose claims concerning what issues will be temporarily honored. (1959)

UNDERGROUND CONVEYORS

The use of underground conveyors to displace confused elderly is an alternative to impression management. Stations employ displacement strategies that are obviously outside of, or in conflict with, clinical definitions of discharge and referral. One underground approach taken is to conceal an encounter, and route the undesirable admission to another similar station: "Once an old man came in a taxi wearing a johnny and an overcoat. The johnny had a Claiborne General Hospital label on it. We called them, and they said they had no record of him having been there. It was obviously a lie" (psychiatric nurse 3, emergency room, CH).

Controlling street transportation, and thereby determining actual bodily presence (or absence) of the person, influences routing decisions.

We don't like to have elderly from the community or nursing homes come in even for evaluation, because once they're here, they're almost certain to be admitted. (psychiatric resident 3, CSH)

Last night we had a confused elderly lady in the emergency room. They referred her to Central State. I took her over, introduced her to the doctor, and said good-by as fast as I could. If the patient's in their building, then she's their problem. (psychiatric nurse 1, emergency room, PH)

If I hadn't put him [an elderly gentleman] in my car and driven him over to the state hospital myself, we never would have gotten him out of here. (psychiatrist 1, CH)

Because medical hospitals do a volume placement business with nursing homes, they are able to place less desirable patients by "making a deal": "If a nursing home accepts a difficult patient from me, I always thank them, and tell them I'll remember them the next time I have a less difficult patient" (social worker 1, CH). One nursing home administrator confirmed this, and reported using the same underground mechanism: "Sometimes I call a place and tell them I'll send them a bad one now and promise a good one later. The placement agents from the hospital make the same deal with me" (head nurse, Holst Nursing Home).

This bargaining is advantageous, since otherwise unacceptable patients can be discharged from the hospital and placed in a nursing home. What effect, if any, this has on the patient's length of stay in the nursing home is questionable. Protecting its relationship with the referral source is one incentive for a nursing home to keep the patient. The home, however, may be able to remove the troublesome patient by making the same deal with another home. The home may discharge the resident to another medical or mental hospital in hopes of filling the bed with a more cooperative patient.

Blacklisting is another underground mechanism influencing the movement of confused elderly. Although its use is generally denied, medical and mental hospitals have identified inferior homes.* The deliberate use of homes known to be inferior is an option for placing the least desirable elderly. Homes that have problems securing admissions from placement organizations because of their bad reputations may be offered patients that "better" homes refuse to accept. That such arrangements exist is evidenced by Central State Hospital's choice of a home that the geriatric specialists considered inadequate and Public Hospital had blacklisted (see Chapter 5). Also, according to welfare worker 2, professionals deliberately inflict future punishment on disruptive and burdensome patients by placing them in inferior and punitive nursing homes.

ORGANIZATIONS AND RESOURCES

Popular knowledge and sociological wisdom attribute to organizations a survival imperative (Etzioni 1961; Kirk and Greenley 1974). The quest for resources is a major factor influencing an organization's exchanges with its environment. Participants (patients and/or clients) are an essential resource for human servicing organizations. At a minimum, patients provide a rationale for their existence. Participants are also liabilities. Organizational resources are spent when services are consumed. Therefore, agencies strive to control their exchanges with participants in order to maximize assets and minimize liabilities. A patient or client who brings more liabilities than assets to the organization is a poor candidate for admission. This section examines the resource quality of confused elderly as organizational participants. Quality is defined in terms of economic and social variables employed by professionals to measure an individual's assets and liabilities (see table 8).

Liabilities

In some stations all confused elderly are perceived as economic liabilities. With the escalating costs of medical care and hospitalization, social agents and

---

*Blacklisting remains an underground activity because continuing care workers often witness unverifiable events and lack sufficient accumulation of evidence to bring formal charges. The workers fear that open discrimination against a home without adequate evidence would have undesirable political repercussions for the hospital.

TABLE 8
Resource Quality of Confused Elderly

Liabilities	Assets
Economic	
Unqualified consumer	Filling a bed
Excessive consumption	Third-party payment
No reimbursement	Pensions
Social	
Disrupt order	Symbiotic relations
Lower morale	Tooling
Besmirch reputation	

the public are sensitive to unnecessary expenses. Admitting officers regard admission of the confused and dispossessed as unwarranted expense: "We must do a physical exam on every admission. . . . The total cost would come to between $300 and $800 for someone who really doesn't need medical care" (medical resident 3, CH). Confused elderly are also defined as economic liabilities when it is perceived that they use a disproportionate amount of a station's resources.

> They consume a great deal of staff time just for custodial care. (psychiatric nurse 9, CSH)

> For an administrator, Margie is a real pain in the ass. She takes a lot of time and staff resources. (chief resident, Service A, CSH)

Manipulating the financial responsibility is a major incentive in routing confused elderly. Prior to Medicaid legislation, the federal government had not contributed directly to the support of persons in mental hospitals. Residents were maintained at the state's expense. Then the aged in these institutions became eligible for medical assistance through Medicaid. But in order to qualify for this federal sharing, the state had to demonstrate the use of suitable community alternatives to the mental hospital. Community mental health centers and nursing homes were two specific services the state had to develop. Therefore, states were able to reduce their own costs significantly by discharging hospitalized elderly and placing them in nursing homes (Thompson 1969).

> What we're really doing is passing people back and forth between budgets. It's just passing the buck. (continuing care worker 2, CSH)

> No one wants to pick up the tab. (psychiatric nurse 1, emergency room, PH)

Obtaining Medicaid coverage for a confused elderly person is an important function of the placement organization. If Medicaid clearance is delayed, a hospital may be forced to hold a patient for an unusually prolonged period or to undertake short-term financing of an alternative placement. The results can have adverse consequences for confused elderly. One elderly lady who was described as the "sanest person on the service" had been in Central State Hospital for over two years because of a financing problem (see Chapter 6). Her present situation is only an extension of obviously inadequate financial arrangements made prior to her arrival.

When a general hospital wants to get rid of a patient, they'll sometimes guarantee payment to a nursing home even though Medicaid has not been approved. The guarantee may be for a week or a month. When that time expires, the nursing home must find payment elsewhere. One patient in the hospital was discharged to a nursing home with one month guaranteed payment. When that month expired the patient paid for one more month, and then refused to pay any more. The nursing home promptly discharged her to a mental hospital (welfare worker 3)

Some medical hospitals are accused of displacing patients whose third-party payment expires: "When a patient's insurance coverage expires, the private hospitals send them here. You see it all the time, and it's not right. There's no continuity of care" (psychiatric social worker, CH).

Confused elderly are thought to be social liabilities if they lower the morale of other participants. Whether they are identified as graceless or disruptive or beyond help, morale is enhanced by minimizing encounters with such undesirables.

How can I eat my lunch, and sit next to someone who smells like that? (senior citizen 3)

Of course, the incentive is for us to place patients we don't like. (social worker 1, CSH)

The most obnoxious behavior is the old people defecating all over the place. That's much worse than even physical struggles. (psychiatric nurse 12, CSH)

Confused elderly are social liabilities when they are thought to besmirch the reputation of a station. The presence of the "irreversibly demented" is a threat to the rehabilitative ideology of the new mental hospital: "Her problem is dementia. She's senile. You ask why we don't help her? Well, there's nothing we can do!" (psychiatric resident 7, CSH). A station's reputation is at stake if confused elderly physically or symbolically disfigure the appearance of the organization.

This place wouldn't look so bad if the old people didn't create such disorder. (social worker 1, CSH)

She won't comb her hair. She won't wash. She goes out in the cold with sneakers and a sweater. Then the neighbors give us a hard time. She really puts you over a barrel when she does that. (staff nurse, Bank Nursing Home)

A nursing home cannot admit "too many" ex-patients from the state hospital without acquiring a bad reputation: "We usually take no more than a third from state hospitals because the home will get a reputation, and then the general hospitals will no longer send their patients" (nursing home administrator, Thompson Corporation). The significance of a good reputation is evidenced by the placement organizations' practice of blacklisting homes identified as inferior. Blacklisted homes will have a harder time filling their beds and are therefore likely to lose money.

Assets

There are economic advantages to handling confused elderly. Level-three nursing homes, the most frequent placement resource for confused elderly, are reimbursed by federal and state governments under medical assistance and Medicaid legislation. By keeping their beds filled, nursing homes can maximize income. The effect of financial incentives on admission decisions is illustrated below:

In the beginning I got the worst ones, but when you have empty beds. (head nurse, Court Nursing Home)

I get angry with homes that will take anyone just to fill a bed. (social worker, Veterans' Hospital)

Families, like institutions, are responsive to economic incentives.

My friend won't put her husband in a nursing home even though the doctor keeps insisting on it. If she does, she'd lose her husband's $108 a month from the Vets and $269 a month pension. She lose all that money to the nursing home, and have to go on welfare. (senior citizen 6)

There are some noneconomic benefits to be realized in handling confused elderly. Social agents and participants enter symbiotic relationships. A psychiatric resident at Central State Hospital made his decision to treat an elderly lady on the basis of her potential contribution to his practice (see Chapter 8): "She's a major community resource! She could help me place my patients, so

I offered her a job. It's a barter. I help her, and she helps me" (Psychiatric resident 10, CSH). Confused elderly sometimes have complicated medical problems, and teaching hospitals need patients with interesting diseases or injuries. Research hospitals use patients as subjects. Even elderly patients in the mental hospital recognized this implicit exchange in the organization-patient relationship.

> I'm in a dream experiment. They're recording my brain waves. I don't like going to bed at night with all those wires on me. Maybe if I felt better I wouldn't mind. I may be helping them, but they aren't doing anything to help me. There isn't any treatment. (Simon, patient, CSH)

There is evidence that professionals find ways to transform potential liabilities into assets. This practice is identified in the field as "tooling" patients for the staff's benefit.

> [In spite of a recent psychiatric consultation in the nursing home, a confused resident was brought to Central State Hospital by the home administrator. The admitting officer analyzed the situation this way]: This is a vendetta against the psychiatrist by the home administrator. [The consulting psychiatrist did the intake evaluation on the administrator two years ago when he was a patient in the hospital.] The administrator is using the patient to complain about the quality of the psychiatrist's service. It's a good example of how patients are tooled. (psychology intern, CSH)

> We found a way of striking back at the VA. His family kept calling us five times a day. So we told them we didn't know if we could keep him, but we were sure that the VA hospital could, so they should get on the phone and talk to them. It worked. We haven't heard from them since, and the VA is now evaluating him. (psychiatric resident 11, CSH)

Confused elderly are rarely accepted as desirable patients, clients, or residents. Their liabilities to servicing organizations usually outweigh their assets. The frequency of their movement on the loop is related, in part, to the extent of their liabilities. Some individuals with a positive asset to liability ratio escape the looping pattern. The nature of defined assets varies according to the station, but confused elderly who are docile, not disruptive, who have Medicaid or personal wealth, and who demonstrate deference and gratitude increase the likelihood of acceptance at any station.

IMPLICATIONS FOR
RESEARCH AND
PROGRAM PLANNING

RESEARCH

The beginning of applied social research is the identification of social problems. To select a problem for study implies that it can be ameliorated through changes in social policy, new programs, or resource reallocations, and that the research can be related to ameliorative strategies. The following five topics are extracted from the Claiborne data and developed as researchable social problems: the family and the social agent, the right to intervene, consultation as a social encounter, a definition of responsible medication practice, and quantitative measurement of discharge planning.

The rediscovery of the family unit suggests to social scientists that they have understimated its true maintenance potential. The family is sometimes described as a natural support, which implies it has a unique and significant role. It is popular to expand this point of view to say that it is morally and economically good for social agents to maximize, within realistic limits, family participation in handling elderly parents, particularly confused parents. According to this model, a cluster of family members, concerned social agents, and perhaps the parent would all work together to achieve mutually satisfactory maintenance solutions. Evidence is presented that such a conception is unreal. In fact, hospital staff describe participating families as uncooperative when they object to hospital plans, particularly about discharge. For the staff to encourage family participation would be synonymous with encouraging conflict. Since community maintenance resources for confused elderly are both few in number and in ill-repute, any placement decision is likely to be viewed unfavorably by an actively participating family. When the dialogue becomes a conversation that tolerates the parent's self-expression of personal preference, the decision making becomes significantly more complicated.

The following questions might be submitted to a research inquiry: In what decisions do social agents inhibit or discourage family participation? How do they do it? In what decisions do families have a stake and assert their interests? When decisions must be made by negotiating incompatible interests, what forces can one set of actors bring to bear against the other? To whom does the greater social power belong? How often and under what circumstances are supposedly senile parents invited to participate in decision making? How much power do they have to influence outcomes? Under what conditions, and about what issues, can mutually satisfactory decisions be made?

The social agent's right to intervene and alter the life circumstances of individuals, without their permission or in spite of their objections, is a major social policy controversy. The citizen's right to privacy, and mental hospital patient's right to treatment, recently have developed into national political issues. The rhetoric of democracy emphasizes the importance of the individual's rights and freedoms. Certain social agents, however, are licensed by society to usurp those rights under special circumstances. Does the physician have the right to deliver the best medical care available, just as the patient has the right to refuse treatment? When the individual is labeled senile or demented, how does the social agent balance the obligation to protect against an obligation to respect the individual's rights?

Obviously, this is an issue not readily submitted to empirical inquiry. The problem was encountered in several settings in Claiborne. An elderly lady was convinced by a psychiatric resident to come to Central State Hospital for an "evaluation," and upon arrival was committed. A confused elderly apartment dweller was admitted to the medical hospital for observation after a fall, and later discharged to a nursing home without ever being told she was not going home. The problem of protective custody versus personal freedom in the nursing home has been analyzed. In each case, questions can be raised about institutional needs, professional assessment, and patient rights. Collecting histories of such incidents in handling confused elderly and sorting them out according to some conceptual framework might prove to be a valuable exploratory investigation. One possibility is to use the concept of deviant or patient careers and analyze patterns of incidents as stages in career development. The results might be useful in educating and encouraging social agents to think about the problem.

Consultation is an intervention strategy enthusiastically endorsed by community mental health ideology. Yet its application in Claiborne proved to be a problematic format for social encounters. The geriatric specialists in nursing homes would recommend to the staff that someone "get involved" with the problem patient. Besides being too obvious to be helpful, the suggestion could instigate the retort, "Why don't you get involved since you're the specialist?" The consultants' own tacit refusal to act on the advice they give challenged the credibility of their advice and the meaning of the encounter. Consultation in the nursing home without simultaneous commitment to enactment of the proposed ameliorative strategies did not prove to be a viable model. In settings where there was less status difference between consultants and consultees (for example, the medical hospital), consultees were more likely to express open disapproval of the consultant and complain about a lack of thoroughness, interest, and commitment.

These inherent defects in the format of the encounter may have implications for the effectivenes of the model in influencing consultee behavior and patient condition. The situation warrants a more elaborate investigation. Perhaps the problem is unique to cases where the patient is presumed to be senile, but the effectiveness of community mental health consultations might be more generally tested for viability among all kinds of clients.

The use of psychoactive medication is always a controversial issue. The excessive tranquilization of elderly is a concern among geriatric psychiatrists. There have been accusations that medications are pharmaceutical straitjackets. The advocates respond that it is better than existing alternatives, and that medication can be and is responsibly prescribed. There were problems with overuse, but according to advocates, those days are gone.

What are the contemporary social definition of "responsible medication"? It is an interesting subject and challenging research because the social definition itself is in transition. The professional debate revolves around the question, "Who is qualified to prescribe?" The issue is also complicated by a lack of consensus among experts about what medication and what dosage ought to be prescribed for those presumed to be senile. There is uncertainty about clinical indicators of medication need, about deleterious side effects, and about the summative effect of multiple medications. There is another debate of smaller proportion about the need for presumed senile to receive perpetually a maintenance dosage of tranquilizers. Questions are also raised about who monitors the maintenance dosage, how often, and the responsibility of the physician who signs the prescription. Taking these factors into account, the exploratory research question might be: Can an "ideal" profile of medication decisions and procedures be constructed, and if so, what is it?

A second research investigation might construct a profile of "real" medication decisions and procedures, that is, medication as it is practiced in the field. Numerous incidents of medication by negotiation were observed. In the nursing homes, house doctors, psychiatric residents, psychiatric nurses, nurse practitioners, and the head nurses were all part of the act. The head nurse was the most forceful of the negotiators. The physician's role was sometimes only ceremonial. The head nurse could also enforce or subvert any medication decision. In the mental hospital, the staff tranquilizes elderly patients when conditions on the ward generally deteriorate. The decision reflects peacekeeping strategies for the ward, not any change in the elderly patient's behavior. These are social factors that are not usually incorporated into professional accounts of medication practices. It might prove interesting to compare a social factor profile to the ideal profile.

Although discharge planning and aftercare are principles highly esteemed in professional doctrine, and mandated by law, they are erratically carried out in mental and general medical hospitals. Quantitative research could measure the frequency and thoroughness of professional activity in this area. It would require a brief preliminary investigation into the legal mandates, prevailing professional rhetoric, and organizational claims regarding these practices. The Claiborne data suggest that it would be useful to measure patient participation in decision making, preplacement visits, preparation of written aftercare plans, and number of postplacement contacts. Postplacement contacts should be measured in length, substance, and format (personal visit or phone call). Such a study could be supplemented by further inquiry into the organizations's budget and manpower investment in placement and aftercare planning. Investment could then be compared to the need for services as determined by the rate of patient turnover and the resources of patients who constitute the hospital's clientele. It was observed that the investment is very small and inversely correlated with constituency need.

PROGRAM PLANNING

This study has identified what could be called defects in the community response. Apart from the value of knowledge for its own sake, it is important that the accumulation and analysis of facts are useful to the construction of ameliorative strategies.

Simply the presentation of data is useful to social agents. It brings together the highly disparate worlds of social agents and confused elderly. It may provoke a keener interest in and appreciation of confused elderly's survival struggles and stimulate the provision of concrete services to ease the burden of that struggle. Social agents, particularly specialists, might respond with more caution in the use of labels and stereotypes. Because the data clarify domains of activity according to type of station, social agents can better know what contribution to expect from one another. By constructing a holistic pattern, the data give to each station a community and organizational context that few practitioners have an opportunity to construct. Ideally, a better understanding would lead to more sympathetic and less acrimonious exchanges between stations. The specific application of these ameliorative themes to particular stations and agents are left to the special interests of the reader.

The inadequate response to confused elderly is not a minor failing of the community. The defects are intrinsic to the system itself. Practitioners' decisions and organizational actions are premised on the irreversibility of senility and the futility of improving the confused state. Apart from propaganda

addressed to popular culture in general and professional social agents in particular, there is no way to attack such pernicious assumptions. They are too well
integrated into the substance of social reality and the fundamental structure
of the community response. The existing pattern is not an accident. It is the
result of specific societal demands. The pattern is a century old; only the
format changes. The possibility of an enlightened redefinition of senility being
generated from within the existing establishment is very slight. Contemporary
community care and the history of institutional care for these elderly are
pathetic. The traditional options forecast a bleak outlook for the future. The
evidence points to a need for a new service structure, one that does meet daily
survival needs without challenging existing doctrine and is complementary to
existing stations.

AN ALTERNATIVE PROPOSAL: A DISCUSSION OF GOALS, SERVICES, MANPOWER, IMPLEMENTATION, FINANCING AND BUDGET, AND RESEARCH

Goals

Individual goals include: identify confused elderly who face impending
relocation, provide survival-oriented service that will stabilize life circumstances and reduce mental confusion, and preserve the individual's community
integration. Goals for the Community are to reduce the total number of
disposition transfers within the community and to reduce interorganizational
antagonism.

No one in the community systematically provides basic survival services.
As a result, confused (and other) elderly are unnecessarily displaced from one
station to another. The proposed strategy would intervene at the crucial stage
of transfer, at the moment when confused elderly are in motion on the loop.
There are obvious advantages to earlier intervention and prevention, but outreach is complicated and produces small returns for large investments. Program resources would be concentrated in direct service delivery to those whose
situation is already seriously deteriorated. Such persons do exist, and in large
numbers. A public general medical hospital could provide access to them.

It is expected that services would reduce mental confusion and improve
situational stability. Basic concrete needs for shelter, food, clothing, safety,
conviviality, and independence are the most persistent and demanding of the
confused elderly's daily experiences. Decline is partially a result of the inability
of the individual to satisfy these needs and the absence of appropriate supportive mechanisms. The proposed program would offer concrete survival assistance, and the service emphasis would be on dirty work. At an extreme, the

program would accept total management and maintenance responsibility for a limited period of time. Without this clearly defined responsibility, the program would have a built-in incentive to discriminate against the most complicated and time-consuming cases. Ideally, medical stations could be convinced to reciprocate for benefits derived from program activity. If so, the program could efficiently and effectively handle treatment, management, and maintenance responsibility on a temporary basis.

The objective of environmental stability presumes that there is greater benefit for the confused elderly in recovering the present situation than in routing and relocation. It should be recognized that extreme circumstances could negate that assumption, for instance, if a neighborhood is absolutely unsafe, if a nursing home abuses a resident, or if the individual wants a residential change. Also, reducing the number of transfers should not be confused with discouraging discharge from stations to private residences. In fact, the proposed program would provide services to support that move.

To preserve existing community integration of the individual, if any, would be another program goal. Confused elderly in transition may lose their apartments and furnishings and their personal possessions and clothing. The program would seek to safeguard property and maintain the individual's permanent residence, whether a nursing home bed or apartment. The cooperation of natural supports, a participating family or friendly neighbor, would be cultivated. The program would take responsibility for initiating street experiences, for example, shopping, attending senior citizen centers, and socializing in the park and at the library.

The program would reduce the number of transfers between stations. As a community strategy, it ought to alter human traffic patterns on the whole loop. It would not be possible to observe or measure the sum of direct and indirect benefits experienced by all loop stations. Measurable benefits would accrue, however, to centralized routing stations. The number of confused elderly admissions would be significantly reduced, and discharge and placement would be facilitated. Although the timing of admission and discharge is always a problem, this program would provide routing agents with a more flexible time frame.

Services

To accomplish the proposed intervention strategy, program personnel must be on duty 24 hours a day, seven days a week. Otherwise the program would be seriously handicapped. The most difficult routine problems occur at night, on weekends, and during holidays when regular servicing stations are closed or minimally staffed. A 24-hour-a-day-operation would also lend the program visibility and conspicuous utility among the existing community stations.

The program is to be oriented toward doing what was previously defined as dirty work in the community. The substance of dirty work was elaborated in the data presentation, but it is useful to review the basic dimensions. The provision of immediate shelter with supervision is the keystone of the initial intervention and subsequent action. When a routing action is being contested, the conflict is usually associated with the timing of the displacement. A short-term shelter for the confused elderly in question would give the discharging station immediate relief and the receiving station an opportunity to prepare alternatives if necessary. Immediate shelter would also serve confused elderly who are discovered in the street or in a state of extreme functional deterioration. To supply such a service, the program would have to maintain a number of beds, determined by the size of the community and the investment in the program. Beds plus supervision could be retained by reserving level-three nursing home beds or rest home beds or by maintaining a small-scale boarding house.

Preferably, short-term boarding would not result from the initial encounter. Rather, the confused individual would be escorted back to the place of residence, whether private or public, and immediate action taken to resolve the situation precipitating the transfer action. At a minimum, an on-site visit to the residence and investigation would be made. Boarding could be considered after the investigation was completed. At the time of intervention, workers would immediately collect detailed life situation data and present it to routing agents, who would use this information in their decision making.

Once a confused elderly individual came under the auspices of the program, daily face-to-face contact for a minimum of a two-week period would be standard procedure. If the individual were in a private residence, the worker would be responsible for organizing personal finances, apartment hunting, supplying food, preparing meals, house cleaning, trash removal, and home maintenance. Local escort service would be provided for shopping, recreation, doctor appointments, and so on. Obviously, a substantial portion of the worker's time would be spent in street transit. It is important that time on the street be recognized as a legitimate program expenditure. Certainly the program would be organizationally concerned with efficient and economic means of transportation, but there would be no program policy to minimize time in transit.

Program workers would take responsibility for securing additional assistance—medical care, dental care, home health care, visiting nurse service. If they could not procure the additional services judged necessary, final obligation would belong to the program either to finance or provide those services directly. As a result, there is both an incentive to do what is necessary to stabilize the individual's life situation and for fiscal responsibility. Nursing home placement or transfer is one activity the program would not undertake. There are significant economies of scale in the placement enterprise. This type of program could not perform the placement function with the same efficiency as the large-scale placement organizations in the general medical hospital. Rather, the program would rely on the cooperation of the participating hospitals to do placements.

Manpower

Only persons without professional credentials would be hired to work directly with confused elderly, since they would not be previously indoctrinated in the rhetoric of senile dementia and organic brain syndrome. They would be less likely to have acquired ideas about "unremittable, irreversible" mental illness. According to professional standards, the job would be primarily menial labor. Depending on the unemployment rate among human servicing professionals, there would probably be few job applicants with professional credentials anyway. While it might be more idealistically democratic not to discriminate against education, it is to the program's advantage to do so. Even professionals who are willing to take menial jobs are not likely to stay for long. In Claiborne, job perseverance among nonprofessionals was greater than among professionals. Also, professionally trained persons who take their education seriously would no doubt discover opportunities to apply their expertise. The dirty work emphasis would be vulnerable to professional distraction. It would, however, be potentially expedient to hire professionals for ceremonial roles. For example, a physician figurehead would lend credibility to the program among community stations.

Would anyone take the dirty work job in this program? The work is unsavory. There are minimal personal rewards intrinsic to the job. Being on the street at any time, day or night, is dangerous. In order to provide 24-hour-a-day service, employees would be required to be on call for emergencies. Staff salaries are a large part of any program budget, and significant economies are to be expected by hiring nonprofessionals. Hiring anyone to do the dirty work would require, however, a salary compensation. Noncredentialed workers would be less expensive than professionals, but not inexpensive employees.

With what discipline or organization should workers be identified? Community maintenance of confused elderly could be categorized as a community mental health program, a public health program, a visiting nurse-homemaker program, a continuing care unit program, or a medical social services program. The proposed model resembles more closely public health and visiting nurse strategies than any other. It remains an open question.

The number of staff would be determined, in the beginning at least, by the size of the program budget. The number should be flexible in order to compensate for fluctuations in demand for service. The flexibility could be accomplished through an on-call policy for regular employees and the use of auxiliary employees. For example, licensed practical nurses could be hired on short notice to supervise the maintenance beds during periods of greater use.

Implementation

The success of the program would be contingent upon establishing complex interorganizational associations. A large number of stations would be involved; routing is complicated and prone to conflict. It is to the advantage of the program to be doing a job that no one else is doing, but which everyone wants done. All this assumes successful service delivery, community visibility, and proven reliability. For example, the general medical hospital staff must be convinced that the confused elderly in the emergency room would be competently supervised elsewhere. Even though the hospital would be informed of the program's role as an alternative to admission, knowledge alone would not alter existing patterns. It would be necessary for a program worker to make regular appearances in the emergency room and to intervene with appropriate confused elderly arrivals. The police and fire departments would likewise be cultivated by regular appearances at the precinct headquarters and the fire station houses. The cooperation of maintenance and residential settings would require more thorough cultivation.

Program success would also depend on enlisting the active participation of stations that benefit from program services. For example, the police, who are frequently involved in transporting confused elderly, would be expected to protect night workers who are on the street because of a routing emergency. Failure of the program to stabilize the confused elderly person's present environment might necessitate nursing home placement. Prompt action by a hospital placement organization would be essential because the program would not offer long-term residential maintenance. The quick and permanent resolution of routing problems is the ideal. Hospitals that benefit by routing disposition problems out of the institution would be expected to provide prompt medical backup, preferably also outside the hospital, if such service is not already available.

Financing and Budget

In the beginning, the proposed program would have to acquire startup funds, from either public or private sources as an experimental demonstration project. Ideally, some range of delivered services would become reimbursable through temporary exemptions from public financing mechanisms now in existence, such as Medicare, Medicaid, and public welfare. Eligibility would be granted at the state and federal levels for alternatives to present reimbursable services. The proposed exemptions would have political viability owing to the prospect of cost economies or the promise to at least test cost economies. If the program acquired an autonomous service identity apart from mental and medical health service systems, how would it be financed in the long run? Would a new public reimbursement mechanism be necessary or desirable? These are important but unresolved questions that a service demonstration would help to answer.

Time-consuming work, policies regulating daily face-to-face encounter, and a high investment in street transit combine to produce a low case load potential. This would be offset by concentrating staff manpower in direct service. Even though a substantial central administrative staff would be advisable with such a geographically diversified service strategy (for the sake of coordination and quality control), it would be sacrificed to financing direct service personnel. The workers would be expected to function independently with a minimum of supervision and backup. This policy would extend the number of direct services produced and reduce the program's salary expense.

Maintaining the proposed domicile would also be a substantial budget item. The program would pay for a fixed number of "bed" services, whether or not the beds were occupied. It is essential to have this service in reserve for emergency routing problems that result in a short-term or permanent transfer of residence.

The conception of service delivery implies extensive street transit. The program budget would reflect the emphasis. Program implementation would require further exploration of the most economical transportation package. The use of taxis, cars owned by employees, ambulances, a fleet of cars maintained by the program itself, or a mixture of these options would constitute the transportation expenses.

Research

As a demonstration project, the proposed program would have a strong evaluation research component. The two principal evaluative questions would be: Does the provision of concrete survival services stabilize the behavior and the life circumstances of confused elderly in risk of being routed? Are there new economies to be derived from this program in the total public costs of treatment, management, and maintenance? The research strategy would also collect ancillary routing data to which workers would have access as a result of their intervention.

The research component would also play a preliminary role in the formation of the organization and implementation of the program. The research effort would systematically collect and analyze data on the following questions:

Are there people willing to do the kind of dirty work described? Does the nature of the work cause a high staff turnover rate? What are the characteristics of the worker who perseveres? How readily is the program integrated into the community pattern? How long does it take? What are the points of resistance, and how are they overcome? Does the availability of detailed information on daily self-management influence routing decisions? Can the proposed services be made immediately available on demand? What is the minimum centralized administration necessary to coordinate the geographically dispersed workers?

The research component would be responsible for collecting service statistics. Since the proposed range of services is unique, it would be important to collect data on the frequency of each service activity and on the distribution through time of cases encountered. Records would be kept on worker time in transit, time in face-to-face contact with confused elderly, and additional time devoted to case management. Data would indicate what number of confused elderly a worker could be expected to handle. Demand for services would also be related to the demographic characteristics of the aged community being served.

To return to the first of the two principal evaluative questions, what is the effect on routing, the paradigm in Table 9 delineates routing decision variables to be tested in conjunction with treatment variables. Data on these same variables would be collected in a comparison community in which there is no similar treatment program. The second community should be comparable on demographic characteristics of the elderly population, in the number and size of level-three nursing homes and rest homes and in the geographic concentration of elderly ex-mental hospital patients.

TABLE 9

Routing Variables

Independent Problem Definition	Intervening Treatment	Outcome
Disposition		
Environment unknown	Life situation data	Admission
Environment unacceptable		Rejection
Medical		
Requires observation	In-residence service offered	Outpatient treatment, placement
Requires treatment, not hospitalization	Temporary boarding	
Treatment history		Referral to program
Mental hospital		(service statistics)

Case histories would be the primary data source. Histories would be kept from time of initial encounter to one year after termination of services. At critical times and in periodic reassessment, the satisfaction of all participants would also be measured. Reducing emotional conflict associated with dumping is a principal aim of the strategy. The effect of relocation stress on mortality rate is one indicator reported in the literature. It would also be necessary to record changes in extent of confused behavior and to measure the effect of program intervention on such changes. The information would be collected through interviews using structured questionnaires. The same interview process would be used to refine the understanding of routing factors, for example, frequency of specific factors, the relative importance of one to another, and variations according to settings.

The research component would also assess costs of the program and compare costs to benefits. Assigning dollar values to social benefits is, of course, a problem. What is the economic value of reduced conflict or of the confused elderly's improved well-being? As a result, the research would be limited to a cost comparison study. It is assumed that reducing the number of transfers and handling transfers more efficiently would save public dollars. The derived economies can be compared to the costs of the experimental program. Sources of economies would be found in costs associated with transportation (particularly use of ambulances), unnecessary hospitalization and delayed discharge, staff time lost in protracted negotiations of routing decisions, and unnecessary institutional maintenance.

MISSING THE DAILY REALITIES

For confused elderly, those characterized as having few resources and little competence, survival is a struggle of immense proportions. Obtaining food, shelter, safety, medical attention, conviviality, money, and clothing are daily preoccupations. When conventional means are closed or out of reach, deviance is the only alternative. Ironically, it is sometimes an old person's tenacious and ingeniously deviant behavior that makes him or her vulnerable to being labeled weak, disorganized, and incompetent.

Although the dimensions of need differ with environmental circumstances, the magnitude of the struggle is uniformly overwhelming. A nursing home resident may have a warm, dry place to sleep and three meals a day, prepared with punctilious regularity and modest nutritional value, but privacy, restricted life space, money, conviviality, and independence are daily problems. If nursing home staff fear a confused person will wander and get lost, that person is confined to the building. Climbing out a window and down the fire escape at night, for whatever personal reason, is construed to be further evidence of mental incompetence. Such existential realities as personal motive, or the hope of adventure and good times are negated by the deviant dimension of the act. Confused elderly on the street have the advantage of independence, mobility, and expanded life space, but safety, keeping clean, and acquiring money and possibly shelter are overriding daily necessities. If an elderly lady has no place to wash, and therefore smells bad, she will be rejected from the senior citizen center where she could have had a free hot meal. If an elderly gentleman cannot restrain his nonconventional speech and mannerisms, he, too, will be excluded from the conviviality and nutrition provided for seniors.

Under oppressive conditions and without resources, it is no wonder that some confused elderly appear to go to great lengths to satisfy their basic needs. If their circumstances are sufficiently desperate, they must make use of whatever resources exist. From their point of view, it is irrelevant whether the use is conventional or deviant. They are not concerned if their behavior disrupts station routine or worries or outrages social agents. It may be, in fact, the social agents' routine and perspective that precipitate behavior by elderly that is purposely defiant and manipulative. The illustrations appeared in all community settings: the lady who made her home in the hospital emergency room for a week; the man who defied the entire nursing home staff from inside a dumpster; the lady who violently resisted commitment to the mental hospital after being coaxed to the admission clinic under a false pretext; the escapees from the medical hospital and nursing home; the bag lady who bathed at the bathroom sink in the emergency room.

The task of summarizing a large volume of information creates a threat of unreal oversimplification. Taking this possibility into account, complexities that are not conveyed by generalizations will be elaborated. By emphasizing the social context of confused behavior, it might seem to be implied that such a context always exists and is always the genesis of the observed confused behavior. The data do not justify such an inclusive conclusion. Confusion does occur in the absence of environmental provocation, at least to the eye of a participant-observer. Families describe cyclical fluctuations in the degree of confusion manifested by their elderly relatives. Such cognitive and behavioral changes are not correlated with familial-social changes. Certainly there are financially secure confused elderly who are not preoccupied daily with survival struggles.

The neurological equipment of the brain does degenerate with age, more quickly in some than others. Many are convinced that organic degeneration is independently correlated with confused behavior in the elderly. The effect of variations in extent and location of degeneration is not yet understood. Survival struggles, deviance, social isolation, and neurological deterioration are all advanced as reasonable hypotheses of causation. Attempts to attribute the phenomenon to cosmic forces and astrological events are indicative of uncertainty and eccentric speculation. Confused behavior has not been successfully traced to any one cause.

Unfortunately, the survival struggle goes unnoticed by social agents; they are too far removed from the daily lives of confused elderly, witnessing deviant behavior in the absence of any social context. A lack of empirical knowledge about environmental details and about the complexity of the survival struggle is glossed over with glib generalities about the debilitating effect of social isolation and dehumanizing institutions. On a community visit to a nursing home, the mental health consultant acquires only superficial information in a short period of time about a patient's disruptive behavior, a condition that is probably long standing. The consultant may suspect both the staff's veracity and the resident's credibility. However, separating fact from fiction even at a superficial level is difficult, and reconstructing the social context in detail is impossible. An admitting officer in the hospital emergency room may have no idea at all of the patient's community life and circumstances if the patient's speech is incoherent. At best, an ambulance driver or policeman may be a source of sketchy information about events immediately preceding and precipitating the patient's arrival at the hospital.

Barriers to Daily Life Details

Social agents are removed by physical, social, and ideological barriers from the details of the confused elderly's daily life. Their physical removal is discussed in detail in the following section. The social distance between doctors and patients, particularly poverty patients, has long been a popular topic with medical sociologists (Croog 1963).

One function of the institutional setting is to facilitate this difference. In institutions, the power of a social agent over a confused elderly person is at an extreme. Decisions about admission, length of stay, medication, discharge, and future residence are made without the confused elderly's participation, and are sometimes contrary to the client's wishes. The contrast in privileges and amenities allowed to staff and patients dramatizes their social distance. In the community, social agents and elderly participants are aware of the social distance separating them from the confused, and purposely preserve it. Senior center members relegate to a socially inferior position those elderly who fail to meet their middle-class standards of grace and decorum. Their response may be one of benevolence or exclusion, but social distance is not altered.

Of the three, the ideological barrier is the most significant. Social agents perceive pathology rather than survival struggles. Pathology is an epistemological framework, borrowed from the medical model of illness and disease used to identify, explain, and predict the course of mental impairment. The meanings of the identifying labels senile dementia and organic brain syndrome are derived from the model of pathology. The credibility and legitimacy of this perspective are derived from its claims to apply scientific principles. Yet it is precisely as a scientific process that it fails to meet its own standards when applied to the aged. Sophisticated medical technology can empirically demonstrate organic deterioration in the brain, but the inferential cause-and-effect relationship between such deterioration and clinical dementia is not proven. Even their simple correlation is challenged in the medical literature. Further correlation between measurements of the mental status exam and the organic condition of the brain is likewise insubstantial. There is confusion about clinical manifestations of the diagnostic categories.

There is minimal agreement among social agents, whether geropsychiatric specialists or nursing home attendants, about the distinct meanings of the several popular labels. The strongest evidence suggests that the terminology is used as a catchall to identify all kinds of deviant and dependent behavior that cannot otherwise be explained. Again, such use is perpetuated in varying degrees by attendants, nurses, social workers, physicians, and geropsychiatric specialists.

The failure of the diagnosis of senility as a scientific process is neither a popular conclusion nor one widely accepted. Errors in individual diagnosis or the exploitative social use of diagnostic categories are attributed to inadequate training or insufficient education of "some" social agents. The guardian against such misuse and abuse is the well-trained and conscientious specialist. This explanation, however, is not supported by the findings of this study. In fact, just the opposite is true. Nonprofessional social agents—LPNs and nursing home administrators, ward attendants, ambulance drivers, patient advocates, and a few registered nurses—are the ones most critical of the use of senile and related labels. Only they went so far as to actually discourage the use of these labels. Physicians, psychiatric residents, and geriatric mental health specialists are true disciples of the pathological perspective and senile labeling. They are the social agents most likely to recognize, or confirm others' recognition of, "senility," and administer the label. There was never a case observed when the specialist diagnosed nonsenility.

Only a few social agents witnessed and participated in both the social world of the specialist in mental pathology, and of the elderly nonconventional survivor. It is no accident that those who knew both social worlds were those most critical of the artificial subordination of one framework to the other. Because of their unusually broad perspective, their evaluations deserve serious consideration, and should not be dismissed as the minority opinion.

From my point of view, the evidence of unsystematic labeling, uncertain etiology, and unreliable predictions, coupled with widely acknowledged social abuses, logically point to the elimination, not the refinement, of the senile diagnostic process. Some would say this is an exaggerated response. Is understanding the causes of senility unimportant? Should the pathologist not explore all plausible avenues? Ought we to give up hope of treatment by eliminating causes? Even if the pathological explanation could be eliminated as a social factor in perspectives and decisions, what would take its place?

Poverty, delinquency, crime, alcoholism, and racism are social problems. I have defined senility as a social problem, and would add it to the list. It is contended that attempts to unravel and sort out the true causes of these social problems are futile. There is no single causative factor. Their complexities are beyond the scope of a single or multidisciplinary inquiry. The conclusions, if any, of multiple causative investigations could not be readily translated into intervention strategies. There is, of course, always the hope of a fortuitous discovery. If that is to be taken seriously as a rationale for causative investigation, then the question of "opportunity costs" must be raised. How much public money ought to be invested in buying chance discoveries when society "cannot afford" to buy for confused elderly the shelter, food, recreation, and medical attention deemed minimally respectable?

If social agents are not to identify certain elderly as senile or organic brain syndrome, then what terms ought they to use? When "diagnosis" is based on clinical observations, then empirical results should be reported, for example, the patient wanders, is forgetful, is incontinent, is an unstable walker, has confused speech. Families, general practitioners, emergency room staff, and continuing care workers could make decisions on the basis of these observations rather than potentially spurious assumptions about causation. If family members want to place their confused relative in a level-three nursing home, it should be because there are too many problems and too few private resources, not because "there is nothing we can do for him."

The Maintenance of Ideological Barriers

The perspective of pathology imposes on the problem a very narrow definition of social reality. In addition to obscuring the significance of daily survival needs, this perspective cannot claim empirical validation. Nonetheless, the previous appearance of research reports and scientific speculation criticizing the diagnostic process has not eroded professional or public confidence in its basic adequacy. Any acknowledgment of its limitations is invariably accompanied by hopeful speculation about future improvements.

The fact that the pathological perspective prevails as the source of social definition in spite of considerable contradictory evidence warrants further comment. To reiterate, social agents are so detached from daily realities of the confused elderly's lives, and lacking in specific information about the individuals they encounter, that the theoretical generalities of their framework are not contradicted. Also, confused elderly are themselves without economic and social resources to defy the social agents and refute the pathological characterizations of their behavior. Social agents have all the power. They know the theories and control the labeling process. They can commit to institutions elderly who oppose admission and refuse admission to those who request it. They control the length of treatment, even place and term of residence. They control the prescription and administration of medication. That confused elderly resist such control can be construed to be further evidence of their pathology. At a theoretical level, there are few opportunities for the elderly to demonstrate a non-"senile" mentality and even fewer in real life.

Beyond the immediate social factors in the social agent-confused elderly encounter are broader cultural forces that sustain the pathological perspective.

Once any deviant behavior is identified as a recurring social problem, theories are recognized, organizations established, and agents authorized to handle the problem. Whatever the social problem, the intervention strategy is directed at "rehabilitating" the individual offender. It is the interventionists' common faith that the welfare recipient, the alcoholic, the criminal, the juvenile delinquent, and so on can be rehabilitated. Though high recidivism rates are the bane of all social agents, few individual deviants are regarded as beyond help. Common faith also dictates that if an individual or entire population of deviants are not readily rehabilitated, then better theories, more specialists, and greater benevolence will accomplish the required therapeutic advances.

The labels "senile dementia" and "organic brain" syndrome are the only diagnostic categories that define the deviant as totally beyond rehabilitation. Only for such elderly is an assumption of therapeutic failure incorporated into the agents' perspective. Senility is like no other deviant label, and its unique quality serves an explicit social function: the diagnosis legitimizes, with the authority invested in the scientist, the exclusion and removal of old people who constitute a social problem. The empirical pattern is clear: those labeled senile presumably cannot be rehabilitated and therefore need only to be maintained, generally in nursing homes. While society hopes that confused elderly are not ill-treated under maintenance strategies, it demands that they are efficiently and economically removed. If they are "senile," it does not matter where they go.

The forces behind the removal of confused elderly are as clear as the pattern itself. One factor that appears peripherally in this study, and is better documented elsewhere (Rosow 1962), is a cultural orientation that values youth and discriminates against aging. Without detailed elaboration, it is enough to say that the bias against aging is an attitude that social agents incorporate as participants in popular culture. More significantly, when community residents are afraid that damage might be done by forgetful and negligent elderly, they favor removal, make their interests known to social agents, and try to influence the agents' actions. The community has an interest in preserving social order. Confused elderly whose lifestyles are disruptive to the middle-class notion of community peace and tranquility are under pressure to be removed. Families often seek relief from maintenance burdens they consider excessive, but are ambivalent about nursing home placement. To displace a parent labeled senile and beyond help resolves the family's conflict and eases the guilt of rejection.

For a professional with esoteric skills, treating confused elderly is not very interesting work. Handling the host of daily maintenance problems is menial labor and too time consuming. Removing confused elderly to a nursing home is an easier solution. The student physician and student psychiatrist want to treat the complex medical and psychiatric impairments. To the student, the confused elderly are usually uninspiring and noneducational patients. Treating them is time not spent in advancing their professional education. The interests of the community and social agents are significantly advanced by defining confused elderly as beyond rehabilitation.

To summarize, it is argued that confusion can be characterized and explained as nonconventional behavior intended to satisfy daily needs. From the social agents' point of view, the confused elderly's behavior is pathological, not ingenious. Social agents do not witness, and are unwilling to intervene in, the daily life details of confused elderly. Those with few resources, inferior social status, and no social power do not successfully oppose senile labeling. When society's needs and the confused elderly's interests are in conflict, societal interests prevail.

The reader might erroneously conclude that the socially inferior and resourceless confused elderly are always at the mercy of self-serving social agents. Social agents—hospital doctors, welfare workers, nursing home attendants—command limited resources, but encounter large numbers of patients with pressing needs. It is a difficult situation. The social agents are committed to their roles and take the performance of their duties seriously. They are frustrated and burdened when they want to help, but cannot. They are conscious of the far-reaching effects their decisions may have on the life of a confused elderly person. When the client's preferences are openly incompatible with the social agent's sense of professional responsibility, the resultant conflict is emotionally traumatic for all participants.

It is also true that social agents do not always prevail. There are confused elderly who successfully use social agents and stations in the most nonconventional ways to meet their survival needs. Institutional staff are pushed to the point of outrage in trying to contend with them. Some confused elderly are identified as con artists because they continually exploit for their own interests the social agents' good intentions. The confused elderly's threats of complaint or promises of recommendation to the stations' administrations have also influenced the actions of practitioners. Even the most down-and-out confused elderly have won victories from their ruling class.

NO STREET ASSISTANCE

There are more confused elderly in the community today than 20 years ago. Mental hospitals have discharged large numbers to "the community," and refused admission to others who previously would have been admitted. To the extent that nursing homes are in "the community," they contribute a large number of elderly officially diagnosed senile dementia or organic brain syndrome. Community residents talked about the sudden influx of confused elderly when the state hospitals began discharging patients in large numbers. There has been, however, no corresponding movement of social agents into the community.

It is useful to interject a comment about the nebulous concept of community. There is a wide-ranging theoretical debate about the true definition of community. Without wading into that debate, it is proposed that access to "the street" is a minimum operational criterion for being considered in "the community." By this is implied that the individual is to some extent free of agent management and can choose independently how to spend the day—where to go and what to do. This best captures the concepts of reintegration and natural supports fundamental to the community movement. According to this criterion, are nursing home residents in the community or in a small-scale institution? For some confused elderly, the nursing home is board and room, and for others it is a way of life. Residents who spend their days on the street are at least minimally in the community. Residents who never leave the home are not in the community. By this definition, the nursing home can be distinguished from the medical and mental hospitals where patients inside the station are not potentially on the street. Other confused elderly who live in private residences or literally on the street are also in the community.

In concert with the notion of community, I propose that the success of "community maintenance work" be measured according to the advances made in the confused elderly's street life. Transferring elderly from the state mental hospital to the nursing home is community maintenance work in appearance only. Applying professional training and psychoactive medication to the achievement of coexistence between distraught nursing home staff and discontent residents does not meet the minimum criterion for doing community work.

Confused elderly are concentrated in nursing homes. This setting would seem to be a logical location for those who aspire to do community maintenance work, but, in fact, it is extremely rare. In Claiborne, only one social agent was observed, the nursing home organizer, who routinely organized street experiences for nursing home residents. For nursing home staff, the routine management of the home does not include regularly escorting residents on the street. The scope of their operation is limited to the physical boundaries of the home and its property. There were two exceptions. A resident could occasionally convince a staff member to supervise a trip to Main Street in order to go shopping and there were also recreational excursions in which all residents were transported to a specific site of entertainment. These were special events, not related to daily routine or local street life. Beyond this, any activities that foster life outside the home, the staff regard as valuable, but a luxury that they can rarely afford to accommodate.

The contribution to street life made by nursing homes is meager, but by other stations it is nonexistent. Senior citizen centers certainly do not solicit membership in nursing homes. Medical and mental hospitals that place their patients do not send their staff to help. Tolerant businessmen and courteous neighbors do more to enhance the confused elderly's street experiences than do the social agents. The nursing home is popularly (and deservedly) subject to intense criticism. If these homes were judged, however, by standards set by the attitude and performance of physicians, nurses, and social workers, the homes would receive superior scores.

For confused elderly in private residences, managing the street is even more complicated, but concrete assistance is again rare. The family is the principal source of help, but at some point, family resources may be exhausted by the maintenance burden, and it is unable or unwilling to continue. Reliance on the family, even if present and cooperative, is a temporary solution. Community work that sustains continuation in private residences, with or without family participation, is complex, very demanding, and time consuming. It involves such aspects as preparing legal, welfare, and Medicaid documents; purchasing groceries and household supplies; preparing meals; feeding the cat; maintaining and repairing homes, from price shopping for exterminators to trash removal; teaching personal hygiene and the management of personal finances; and mollifying angry or anxious neighbors. Beyond this routine maintenance, social agents encounter confused elderly who for a prolonged period have mismanaged or not managed their environment. Retrieving them from the midst of filth and physical deterioration is an unpleasant job. None of the social agents want to do it; most refuse to do it. This is dirty work and menial labor for professionals.

The same absence of community work is apparent in the movement of confused elderly from the community through institutions and back to the community. Elderly who arrive at the medical or mental hospital because of confusion are, in most cases, processed through the emergency room. Unfortunately, the Emergency Room is not equipped to obtain the information about community circumstances that the staff considers necessary. Besides the patient, the only source of outside information might be a police officer or ambulance driver. Admission decisions are made without such useful information as the availability of formal or informal assistance at home and the person's degree of success at surviving in the community prior to appearance at the hospital. There is no attempt to reestablish at home a candidate rejected by the staff. Hospitalization may not be the optimal treatment, but it is the only realistic alternative in the absence of home supports.

When the hospital is ready to return a confused patient to the community, the placement worker tries to locate an available nursing home bed. When a placement agreement is reached between a hospital and a nursing home, the patient goes. Patients may arrive with or without transfer papers and aftercare plans. Continuing care units in the medical hospitals are so understaffed that all direct contact with the patient is terminated at the time of discharge. There is no regular follow-up. Transfer is abrupt; there is no systematic preparation for the confused patient or the home. A greater percentage of confused elderly discharged from the mental hospital will be "visited" in the nursing home, but only at the home's request. Hospital staff follow-up on management problem discharges in order to avoid rehospitalization. There is no "treatment" for nursing home placements. Rarely do confused elderly make their way to a private residence after leaving the mental hospital. If they do, it is on their own initiative. The only geriatric specialty team in the community disavows any responsibility for direct rehabilitative association with confused elderly for whom they are responsible. The organizational components of the central routing stations either will not or cannot, because of skeleton staffing, directly contribute concrete help in the community.

Community work that is addressed to concrete needs is unappealing to social agents. Professionals have trained for more esoteric interventions, and want to employ their special expertise. The few professionals who have been drawn into community maintenance work, experience conflict over their sense of personal responsibility and their professional identity. They do it not because they want to, but because they cannot find anyone else to do it. It seems unconscionable to them to neglect the task.

Only the social agents who are themselves on the street become witnesses to and participants in meeting daily needs. Other social agents, who are stationed in institutions but make occasional forays onto the street, are out of touch with daily realities. Their infrequent and brief interventions are irrelevant in the context of survival needs. They are much more apprehensive and awkward in their performance and obviously unenthusiastic about the task. These agents also have station maintenance responsibilities. Time spent in the community (particularly time in transit) is defined as time lost to the institution. The visibility and immediacy of institutional needs overshadow community needs. The "community workers" employed by institutions cannot afford to advocate community interests that are in conflict with their employers' interests, and therefore tend to represent the institution in the community.

Barriers to a Social Niche

There are also barriers inhibiting the movement of confused elderly from the community to the stations. Every station has a limited supply of resources and faces the specter of unlimited demand. The social power to discriminate among all applicants and selectively admit is essential to the organization's survival. By manipulating the size and character of the beneficiary population, resources are extended in a way that maximally rewards the organization. Confused elderly consume too many resources and offer too few rewards, so they are subject to exclusionary practices. Treatment stations erect barriers to confused elderly because they are defined as beyond rehabilitation. Therapeutic resources invested in confused elderly would be wasted. Maintenance stations erect barriers to confused elderly because they wander and get lost and disrupt the order of the institution. Geriatric specialists avoid a deluge of community requests by refusing to treat anyone directly.

As a result, confused elderly are processed through a series of temporarary situations; their route forms a loop of local human servicing stations. Routing problems are the substance of social agent-confused elderly encounters. Routing agents inhibit admission, facilitate displacement, or keep the peace in order to preserve the status quo. In the midst of this motion on the loop, some elderly never locate and settle into a social niche.

The decision to admit, displace, or retain minimally depends on the degree and specifics of tolerance for deviant behavior at each station. When the deviant style coincides with the station's tolerance, and other liabilities are insubstantial, the confused elderly is allowed to settle in. Routing, however, is more heavily influenced by the relative strengths and weaknesses of stations' boundaries. Confused elderly are moved or retained according to the social pressure of interorganizational associations. Weak boundary stations are unable to prohibit the arrival and physical presence of confused elderly. They do not control the social definition of the "true" problem and appropriate treatment. Organizations with greater social power successfully impose their definitions on weaker stations.

Admission, temporary retention, and locating a social niche are products of interorganizational negotiations. Confused elderly alone do not overcome barriers to command the release of resources. However, confused elderly backed by superior social pressure penetrate the boundaries. A stabilized routing pattern is ultimately an equilibrium of competing organizational interests. The fate of the individual confused elderly is an insignificant factor.

CASE STUDY METHODS AND PARTICIPANT-OBSERVATION RESEARCH

The attempt to apply scientific methodology conscientiously to the investigation of social problems has yielded two major research traditions, one quantitative and one qualitative, or statistical and nonstatistical. Contemporary research falls mainly into the quantitative category, and is generally valued as the more "scientific." It most often takes the form of survey research where analysis consists of cross-tabulating the distribution of one trait with the distribution of another. The unit of analysis—the individual, organization, or social process, for example—representing the wholeness of those traits is not part of the analysis itself. For this reason, a distinction is made between trait and holistic research. In the latter, the commonality of traits is qualitatively described in order to preserve the social phenomenon in its entirety (Goode and Hatt 1952).

Apprehending and reconstructing a community's response to encounters with confused elderly is a case study technique. Qualitative data are collected and organized so as to preserve the unitary character of the community response. The response itself is elucidated in terms of the actors' perspectives and actions.

The wholeness of the case to be observed is captured by employing the following research techniques:

Collect a broad array of data, including as many of the relevant and significant facets as possible.

Use economic, political, and psychological sources of data as well as purely sociological. These dimensions will be added when they help to clarify the social relationships being studied.

Apply typologies and indexes so that various traits can be used to characterize the establishment as a whole.

Emphasize process and time. Rather than making observations at two points in time, noting the differences, and inferring the process of differentiation, in this study the process itself is directly observed. The relevant characteristics as they appear in individual and group interaction are recorded (Goode and Hatt 1952).

The word "perspective" designates the manner in which groups of actors organize their observations and structure their ideas about the way things are so that they can define events, make decisions, and take actions. To ascertain the actors' perspectives, the researcher observes everyday actions and notes empirical regularities in events. He tries to reconstruct the definition of the situation used by those who participate in the encounter. The focus is on the description of prior, immediate, and subsequent events, not on causation. The researcher interviews the participants in detail about their perceptions of the confused elderly's problems and about the contribution of their profession. The researcher selects respondents who have the most experience and are best able to communicate their ideas (Selltiz 1951).

ESTABLISHING AND MAINTAINING THE RESEARCH ROLE

The Research Agenda

The case study approach is costly in terms of research time. It is important to define in advance the domain of interest. The researcher can exercise some control over this variable. The degree of concentration and detail of the analysis is fixed by the nature of the inquiry and the researcher's standards of performance. The object of the study is delimited by the conceptualization of the problem and the time and money available to the researcher. One must reconcile the research ideals of problem identification, investigation, and analysis with resource pragmatism.

The nature of the case study demands a very flexible daily agenda. While in the field, the researcher must be willing to go when and where the action is. Length of interviews and extent of observations vary extensively. The researcher must be able to take advantage of fortuitous events, and spontaneous access to otherwise prohibited areas or events must be followed up immediately. On such occasions, waiting for a better day or more convenient time may mean an irretrievable loss of data. A well-organized interviewing agenda for the day or week will probably be interrupted. The researcher must learn the act of breaking (or missing) appointments without giving offense, which is not easy, given the traditionally precarious researcher-practitioner relationship. Time sampling of institutional routine and surveying night life will put the researcher on the street at all hours. For example, the emergency room staff's complaints about nursing home dumps on the weekend and after 5:00 P.M. necessitated some long and unusual hours.

The mechanics of recording and organizing data are very time consuming. Abbreviated notes were made during the interview or observation period and then elaborated in detail as soon as possible after the data-collecting event. Writing up an hour interview might take as much as an hour or hour and a half, depending on the quality and extent of information. The result is that time devoted to recording data cuts seriously into data-collecting time. For methodological reasons, it is desirable to maintain simultaneous relationships with several stations at one time. Regular attendance at each station is essential. If the practitioner sees the researcher's appearance as sporadic and irregular, he may consider it to be unserious data collection and therefore unworthy of his or her involvement.

Where to Begin?

Having formulated the problem and chosen an investigatory design, taking the study into the field is the next step. From the point of view of the outsider trying to get in, community stations are ordered in degrees of organizational complexity, with the Main Street luncheonette at one extreme and the general medical hospital at the other. The more complex the organization, the less permeable the boundary. Research can be delayed for months while waiting for administrators and research review committees to act on a research proposal. The intricacy of the station's approval process is correlated with the probability of being rejected. Encountering delays and setbacks in the beginning is a substantial hindrance and psychologically unappealing.

In spite of this, beginning with the large institutions is the most practical way to secure introductions to the numerous smaller stations. It should be recalled that the design calls for discovering new elements as well as refining known patterns of community response. City Hospital, Public Hospital, and Central State Hospital process large numbers of confused elderly, and therefore maintain extensive organizational associations in the community. They can provide information as to the scope and diversity of stations involved and, if cooperative, help the researcher gain entree. A referral from one of the hospitals gives the researcher credibility in the local setting that contributes significantly to allaying the local social agent's skepticism about the unknown researcher from the outside.

This field investigation was begun in City Hospital and Central State Hospital, as the design of the study made it impractical to begin in the local settings. Also, the only initial contacts were with these institutions through the university. The researcher's initial overtures are likely to be the most sensitive. At City Hospital, for example, attempts to obtain formal administrative approval were blocked because the administrator with that authority was too busy to see me and referred me to his subordinates. Several weeks were lost before formal approval was granted. In the meantime, I began interviewing practitioners through other contacts in the hospital. What I took to be innocuous forays into the institution, however, resulted in excited accusations that I was trying to "sneak in the back door."

It turned out that different units in the hospital related to different administrative elements. After several weeks of "approved" interviewing, I sought entree into the emergency room, and faced a new problem. My original adminstrative approval was not good enough for them. I had to seek higher authority. This posed the threat of being prematurely evicted from the hospital if a higher authority denied the request. In any event, the outside researcher with low status is perpetually plagued with problems of legitimizing authority if he or she doesn't start at the top. On the other hand, starting there may mean unacceptable delays and a greater probability of rejection. It is very useful to first obtain the line practitioner's approval. The researcher can then say to the administrator, "It's OK with them, if it's OK with you." That turns out to be a very effective argument.

A similar problem arose at Central State Hospital where I had been more successful at avoiding administrators and delays. After nearly completing my study at the hospital, I still had not gained access to the admission process itself. The director of admissions never responded to my calls. Eventually one subordinate did, and he recommended seeing the executive director of the hospital. The executive director told me to submit a proposal to the research review committee. But he didn't know the name of anyone on the committee and couldn't tell me who to contact. That direction seemed to be an exercise in certain futility. I finally achieved my purposes by obtaining the name of the most cooperative of the admission team psychiatric residents. At my request, he spoke to the director who had repeatedly refused to answer my calls, and I obtained immediate informal approval.

The low-key, informal approach taken in these settings proved to be successful. The strategy did result in the compromise of one research objective. I was refused access to patients' records in both settings without going through the research review committee. At City Hospital such approval would have been unlikely under any circumstances. Several staff members described the hospital administration as "nervous" about releasing patients' records. At Central State Hospital, some informants allowed me to read patients' records behind closed doors in spite of formal refusal. The gains in efficiency and security and the minimal loss made the compromise worthwhile.

Evasions and Refusals

Once I had chronologically ordered my field entrees and overcome early approval obstacles, I was continually confronted with the unwilling respondent. A few interviewees simply refused to speak to me.

I don't have anything to say about anything. I don't know anything. (fireman)

Policeman 2: Who's he? I'm not gonna talk to him! I don't know him.
   Policeman 1: [aside to interviewer]: If you asked about horses, he would have talked your arm off.

Less direct but nonetheless effective refusals were also made by professionals. For example, one prominent geriatric psychiatrist agreed to see me only if I paid his standard fee for a "session." On the inpatient service at Central State Hospital when I addressed the head nurse, she simply walked away after listening for about 45 seconds. By refusing to grant me a "socially appropriate" refusal, she put my role on a par with the nuisance patients. They, too, are without the right of conversation in addressing staff (Rosenhan 1973). Another technique is to formally grant the researcher access, but to keep him at the margins. For example, only through repeated requests and repeated reassurances combined with my fortuitous presence was I able to observe in process a mental health consultant community visit in the nursing home. Staff agreed, in principle, that I could accompany them to the nursing home, but they would not inform me in advance of the community visit. The "cooling your heels" technique was also successfully used. In one case I waited 90 minutes for a 20 minute interview. A combination of temerity, patience, and good luck is essential under such circumstances.

Confidentiality, perhaps the practitioners' one true sacred object, is also their shield against researchers' inquiries. Under the authority of the Geriatric Specialist Team leader, I was granted entree to the inpatient service of the hospital. There I interviewed patients and staff alike. At the same time, team members were reluctant to take me into nursing homes because I would meet patients and that would violate their right to confidentiality. I interpreted the inconsistency as a front for other reasons the members were unwilling to make public. The nursing home consultation is a less conventional and more precarious service delivery mechanism. Yet team members did not offer uncertainty about their role or lack of confidence in their performance as an explanation for the reluctant concessions.

While the principle of confidentiality is commendable, its credibility is further diminished with profanation by its professional adherents. For example, at a meeting of the geriatric specialists, the team members were speculating about the nursing home personnel's perceptions of their consultation program and the decline in participation. Since I had interviewed a nursing home administrator on the same topic that morning, I volunteered her observations. Immediately the team leader asked me to identify her. (He had previously admonished me about the necessity of confidentiality.) I considered the comment basically neutral, so relented and gave her name. The team leader then accused her of being psychiatrically imperceptive and dull-witted.

The Practicioner-Researcher Relationship

In principle, the researcher's and practitioner's roles are complementary. At the level of face-to-face encounter, their relationship is invariably strained. In the broadest sense, it can be said that the purpose of applied research in social settings is to discover inefficiency and encourage change. There would otherwise be no need for "formative" research. Practitioners, on the other hand, are predisposed to assert their competence, defend their efforts, and maintain the status quo. Furthermore, the researcher brings to the field an entirely different occupational perspective than that of the practitioner (Caro 1975, 1971).

None of the Claiborne social agents was enthusiastic about having a researcher in their midst. Most tolerated it; a few occasionally enjoyed the role of informant. Even cooperating professionals responded to the simplest data-collecting requests with a sense of apprehension.

> Observer: I would like to sit in on your team meetings.
> GST leader: Well, you know, people don't like to be observed. They are concerned about how they may be evaluated, concerned that someone is thinking they aren't doing a good job. This is a staff decision, and I must leave it up to them. I'll present it at the next meeting.

Some who cooperated might have done better to keep me out. I was occasionally embarrassed to be cultivating a social agent's confidence in order to collect what turned out to be damning evidence.

The researcher who persists in spite of others' evasions and his own reservations has several options. The researcher can try to remain in the background as much as possible or set about to cultivate personal relationships with practitioners (Mann 1971). In the first interview, I learned a fundamental rule in approaching the practitioner—to elaborate in detail the usefulness of the study to the practitioner in general and to the interviewee in particular. To neglect this point was to invite criticism and opposition. Just to promise the study results to a participant was often enough to inspire cooperation.

A willingness to engage in interpersonal gimmickry is very useful. This generally involves posing as the practitioner's friend. To carry out this performance, I gave away seedlings in the springtime, and on community visits I transported practitioners without cars. I also took Central State Hospital ex-patients to hospital meetings and drove nursing home staff home after work. I once offered to help a nursing home recreational worker paint her apartment, but fortunately my magnanimity was turned down.

"Conversion" is a technique with which the researcher portrays his assimilation into the culture of the institution (Goffman 1961). In general, it is a matter of taking on the dress and speech of the staff. For instance, in the corridors of the general medical hospital, I wore a V-neck sweater and tie and maybe a sports coat. This is the fashion among medical students and young doctors. Wearing a white lab coat, the uniform for social workers, psychiatric nurses, psychiatrists, or other professional employees without conspicuous status identification, gave my presence on the medical ward the appearance of clinical legitimacy. On one occasion, I accepted an invitation to come to Sunday dinner at the nursing home. This meal as a social event is ascribed religious and ceremonial significance. Since many acquaintances of the home are invited to dinner but few come, I was an "honored guest," and as such, was called upon to "give the blessing." In spite of a personal aversion to public prayer, I quickly converted to the owners' ideals. In light of my previous vague affirmations of the owners' religious principles, a refusal at that point would have exposed me as an "impostor."

If the researcher is willing to take the time and energy to cultivate practitioners, he can more aggressively assert his interests in the practitioners' setting. Not only should the researcher explain what he hopes to accomplish but he must also be prepared to state exactly what cooperation entails. This is often difficult in the beginning if the researcher knows little about the actual functioning of the setting. Under these conditions, the researcher should consider asking for "everything." The practitioners' notion of unacceptable participant-observation research behavior is as ill-defined as the researcher's vague notions about the situational integration in each setting.

VALIDITY, RELIABILITY, SAMPLING

According to the conventions of traditional social research, validity is the congruence between conceptual and operational definitions. Does the data measure what they are supposed to, and are the operations sufficient to encompass the relevant facts? This classical definition, however, has little relevance in this study. It assumes that one reality is verifiable from an objective, rational, scientific point of view. This study presupposes that one man's reality could be another's gross distortion. There are no conclusions by the "objective" investigator that one reality is true and another false. For the purposes of this study, the question of validity becomes, has the researcher reconstructed the social world of the actor as the actor himself sees it? Does the actor have the perspective that the investigator claims he has? And does the reconstructed perspective describe the set of variables that determine the actor's decisions and actions?

The flexibility of the exploratory research design permits validity testing as a part of the research. The investigator is continually reformulating his perceptions of the actors' world, progressively eliminating the extraneous and marginal variables. Repeated observations and interviews provide an opportunity to retest new formulations. Actors themselves are asked to judge the accuracy of the investigator's conclusions. The investigator's successful assimilation into the alien culture documents, at a minimum, a workable construction of the actor's social world.

The concept of reliability refers to the consistency in measurement. Any variation in results must reflect variation in the social world, not inconsistencies in the measurement procedure. The flexibility of an exploratory case study is not conducive to making the customary checks for stability and equivalence. Assessing reliability is even more complicated in this study because a major subpopulation of respondents is labeled "confused." Is it necessary to assume that the reports by "confused elderly" are unreliable? The answer is obviously no. I have defined the label so as to incorporate explicitly environmental contingencies, not just individual mentality. For example, an elderly lady presumed senile is described by one nurse at Central State Hospital as the "sanest" person on the ward. The ex-mental hospital patients in nursing homes can give internally consistent and coherent accounts of nursing home life. There may be nothing within the report itself to discredit its substance. In all settings, the reliability of "confused" respondents is tested by the confirmation of informants who share their social world and by the confused themselves in their more lucid moments. In this study it becomes obvious that the confused mental state is neither perpetual nor totally encompassing.

The impact of instability and inequivalence in measurement can be reduced by an adequate sampling pattern. For example, repeated interviews with the same respondent provide one source of verification. Questions about the social agent's view of his client, of the organization where he works, and of the other stations were asked of as many different types of agent in each setting as possible. The results of each interview served to check the reliability of the others. The breadth of coverage tests the reliability of individual sources of information.

Each of the constituent elements in the community-confused elderly encounter were sampled: social agents who deal with confused elderly, functional groupings of social agents called "stations," Claiborne confused elderly, and events.

Three general medical hospitals were surveyed. City Hospital was selected because it serves a large indigent elderly population that includes the Claiborne area and plays a crucial role in routing confused elderly. Public Hospital became involved since it is the medical backup for Central State Hospital, the community mental health center and mental hospital serving Claiborne. Both are large teaching hospitals. For the purposes of surveying a range of hospital orientations, Community Hospital, a small, private, fee-paying patient hospital was also included. Within the general medical hospital, the emergency room, outpatient clinics, medical ward, and psychiatric services were sampled.

Central State Hospital, a long established training and research hospital and more recently a community mental health center, was the major source of data on mental health intervention strategies. The following components were included: the Geriatric Specialist Team, the inpatient service, and the continuing care unit. Through these sources, data were also collected on admission and discharge practices.

The concentration of confused elderly in nursing homes, and the concentration of nursing homes in Claiborne, were at first thought to pose difficult sampling problems. The formally designated levels of care range from extensive (posthospitalization, Medicare-financed) to custodial. There is also considered to be a diversity in quality of care within levels. The need to represent the variations in levels was eliminated by the mental and medical hospitals' exclusive use of level-three homes for elderly whose primary disability is confusion (as defined in this study). Sampling a range in quality was a more difficult problem. I suspected in the beginning that inferior homes would deny me access, and sampling would be biased toward better homes. To some extent this proved to be true. Generalizations from the data to all nursing homes must be cautiously advanced.

Among the other local stations, one of the three senior citizen centers was selected for extensive observation because of its close organizational ties with Central State Hospital's community mental health center. I interviewed the director of the second center twice, and observed center activities on several occasions. This provided a check on the validity and reliability of data collected in the original setting. Also, by attending community summer events for seniors, picnics and sing-a-longs, I gained a perspective on the nature of some elderly's confused behavior in public and the community, particularly peer group, response. One of the three community health centers in Claiborne was selected. One of the others was newly formed and the third was geographically removed from the nursing home, senior citizen center, and Main Street sites I had already selected. Only one local organization unconditionally refused me access, the Claiborne Mental Health Outreach Team under the auspices of Central State Hospital. While I was unable to observe its functioning as a unit, I did have numerous interviews with its geriatric specialists, and discussed with them their jobs and the unit.

Tables 10, 11, and 12 comprehensively list the study population of stations, social agent by station, and participants (including confused elderly) by station. Within each station an attempt was made to secure a sample of social agents that represented differences in professional training, status in the organization, and job assignment. An attempt was always made to select respondents with the most experience or who were the most analytic in their thinking and best able to communicate their perspective. On the basis of observation and a "respondent-domino" technique, I was able to make informed guesses as to who would be a quality respondent.

The respondent-domino technique is used for initiating contacts with new respondents and new stations. During each interview I asked respondents to recommend to me the names of other participants who met the above qualifications. If respondents were enthusiastic about my investigation, I sometimes asked them to introduce me to the other respondents or to let me use their names when introducing myself. At the level of front-line personnel where my

TABLE 10

Locales of Observation

Central State Hospital (CSH)
City Hospital (CH)
Community Health Center (CHC)
Community Mental Health Center (CMHC)
Community Hospital
Community Service Association
Fire Department
Library
Main Street Luncheonette
Nursing Homes

Autumn	Holst
Bank	Majestic
Brady	Paradise
Clover	Walden
Court	

Police Station
Post Office
Public Hospital
Senior Citizens Center
Welfare Department
Unspecified (private residence, doctor's office, bus)

interviews were concentrated, the most successful tactic was to be able to say, "Mary Jo said I should talk to you." As an illustration, the domino technique produced the following linear chain of referrals: Geriatric Specialist Team leader to geriatric outreach worker to senior citizen director to a vocal and well-connected senior citizen to the head librarian at the local library to the community health center next door. The technique was also useful with participants other than social agents. For example, a senior citizen advised me: "That one over there is a little soft in the head—you know what I mean. She would be a good one for you to interview." (senior worker, geriatric workshop).

Time sampling proved to be a useful technique for enhancing the representativeness of the sample population. I made observations in nursing homes and on the inpatient service at Central State Hospital at different times of the day and on different days of the week. Each custodial institution has daily routines with distinctive tonal qualities. If the researcher disproportionately samples one phase in the daily or weekly routine, the data would not adequately represent daily life. Also, by hanging out in the emergency room at night and on weekends when the setting was busiest, I acquired a great deal of information in a short period of time, and saw confused elderly-social agent encounters in process rather than just hearing retrospective reports.

TABLE 11
Social Agents by Stations

Medical Hospitals

City Hospital
Medical resident 1
Medical resident 2
Medical resident 3
Medical resident 4
Medical resident 5
Medical intern
Physician
Psychiatrist 1
Psychiatrist 2
Social worker 1
Social worker 2
Social worker 3
Social worker 4
Social worker 5
Psychiatric social worker
Student social worker
Patient advocate
Continuing care worker 1
Continuing care worker 2
Community Hospital
Social worker
Nurse
Public Hospital
Psychiatric nurse 1, emergency room
Psychiatric nurse 2, emergency room
Nurse 1
Psychiatrist
Social worker 1
Veterans' Hospital
Social worker
Registered nurse

Head nurse, emergency room
Nurse 1, emergency room
Nurse 2, emergency room
Nurse 3, emergency room
Nurse 4, emergency room
Nurse 5, emergency room
Nurse 6, medical ward
Nurse 7, medical ward
Nurse 8, orthopedic
Nurse 9, medical ward
Nurse practitioner
Psychiatric nurse 1, emergency room
Psychiatric nurse 2, emergency room
Psychiatric nurse 3, emergency room
Psychiatric nurse 4
Psychiatric nurse 5
Attendant, medical ward
Ambulance driver
Guard

Continuing care worker 1
Continuing care worker 2
Continuing care worker 3
Community health worker

Mental Hospital and Community Mental Health Center

Central State Hospital
Chief resident
Psychiatric resident 1
Psychiatric resident 2
Psychiatric resident 3
Psychiatric resident 4
Psychiatric resident 5
Psychiatric resident 6
Psychiatric resident 7
Psychiatric resident 8
Psychiatric resident 9
Psychiatric resident 10
Psychiatric resident 11
Psychiatric resident 12
Psychiatric nurse 1
Psychiatric nurse 2
Psychiatric nurse 3
Psychiatric nurse 4
Psychiatric nurse 5
Psychiatric nurse 6
Psychiatric nurse 7
Psychiatric nurse 8
Psychiatric nurse 9
Psychiatric nurse 10

Executive administrator
Psychiatrist, Service A
Psychology intern
Occupational therapist
Continuing care worker 1
Continuing care worker 2
Social worker 1
Social worker 2
Social worker 3
Social worker 4
Attendant 1
Attendant 2
Attendant 3
Group leader

Geriatric Specialist Team
Psychiatrist (leader)
Psychiatric nurse 1
Psychiatric nurse 2
Social worker

Nursing Homes

Autumn
  Activities director
  Recreation worker
  Attendant
  Remotivation therapist
  Trainee 1
  Trainee 2
Bank
  Staff nurse
  Recreation worker
Brady
  Staff nurse
Clover
  Administrator (Thompson chain)
  Staff nurse
Court
  Head nurse
  Night supervisor
  Staff nurse 1
  Staff nurse 2
  Recreation worker
  Attendant

Holst
  Head nurse
  Staff nurse
  Activities director

Majestic
  Unidentified male attendant

Paradise
  Employee

Walden
  Cook

Private Physicians

Private physician 1
Private physician 2
Private physician 3
Private physician 4

Community psychiatrist
Geriatric psychiatrist

Community Stations

Community Health Center
  Psychiatric nurse 1
  Nurse
  Community worker

Family Counselling Society
  Family counselor 1
  Family counselor 2

Geriatric Workshop
  Leader

Police
  Captain
  Police sergeant
  Policeman 1
  Policeman 2
  Policeman 3
  Policeman 4
  Policeman 5
  Policeman 6

Senior Citizen Center
  Senior citizen center director 1
  Senior citizen center director 2
  Senior citizen center director 3
Welfare Department
  Supervisor
  Worker 1
  Worker 2
  Worker 3
Miscellaneous
  Community mental health sponsor
    of geriatric workshop
  Geriatric social worker
  Community organizer
  Nursing home organizer
  Nurse, VNA
  Post office clerk
  Bus driver
  Librarian
  Fireman 1
  Fireman 2

TABLE 12

Participants by Stations
(those whose observations appear in the paper; CE = confused elderly)

Central State Hospital patients	Nursing home residents
Simon (CE)	Mary
Margie (CE)	Alice
Lisa (CE)	Katie
Cassandra (CE)	Ed
Frank (CE)	Emerson
Betty (CE)	Ella
Allen (CE)	Nellie
deaf lady (CE)	Peggy
Linda	Lizzie
Carl	Blondie
Peter	Patty
Claire	Fred
Lila	Helen
Paul	Unidentified resident 1
Harriet	Unidentified resident 2
Matthew	City Hospital
Senior Citizen Center	Louise
Senior citizen 1	Elderly gentleman
Senior citizen 2	Geriatric Workshop
Senior citizen 3	Senior worker
Senior citizen 4	Street people
Senior citizen 5	Elvira (CE)
Senior citizen 6	Sonya (CE)
Senior citizen 7	Screaming lady (library)
Senior citizen 8	Unidentified lady (CE, bus)
Jerry (CE)	Panhandler
Main Street luncheonette	Unidentified lady with
Customer 1	Salvation Army companion
Customer 2 (elderly)	Unidentified CE lady
Customer 3 (elderly)	Miscellaneous
Customer 4 (elderly)	Family: father (CE)
Chef	physician-son, daughter
	Family member
	Nursing home neighbor 1
	Nursing home neighbor 2
	Nursing home neighbor 3
	Retired nursing home caretaker

INTERVIEW AND PARTICIPANT-OBSERVATION

Detailed interviewing and observation were the primary data-collecting methods. Each makes available to the researcher a specific kind of information, and the strengths of one minimize the weaknesses of the other. During interviews I questioned social agents about their jobs and the organizations, the etiology and manifestations of confusion in the elderly, specific encounters to illustrate their points, and interorganizational relations. Confused elderly were questioned about means for meeting daily needs (food, shelter, money, safety, conviviality, and so on) and the nature and extent of encounters with social agents.

The interviews were unstructured. In the beginning, I experimented with various degrees of structure in an interview guide that would allow me to organize the interview. The respondents' sometimes rambling associations rarely conformed to my predetermined approach. A single illustration of an encounter might reflect all four of the above themes. To insist on a thematically categorized account would have interrupted the development of the story as the actor saw it. While this approach facilitated the interview, it complicated the organization and analysis of data. Exchanging greater reliability through standardization of the interview for less detailed accounts would have been inconsistent with the goals of the study.

The focus of the interviews (excluding situations of simultaneous interview and observation) was on the retrospective accounts of events. There are certain unavoidable limitations with the approach. Respondents tend to give idealized accounts of their own and their station's activity. For example, my inquiry about the use of tranquilizers with "behavior problems" in nursing homes produced the following textbook response from the Geriatric Specialist Team leader: "Medication is always the last thing to think about." Such idealized abstractions are useless for understanding customary practices. Respondents also tend to conceal secret pleasures and secret economies (Goffman 1959). Assuming the frankness of the respondent, the validity of the account depends upon the accuracy of the respondent's memory. Nonrecurring events, events in the distant past, events of little interest, and events difficult to comprehend increase the fallibility of human memory and must be judged cautiously. The method also encourages the informant to formulate rationales and interpretations for the sake of the interviewer that did not exist at the time of the event described and did not influence it. Finally, the interview technique does not tap the respondent's unconscious motivation and unconscious reasoning.

Conducting group interviews is one check on the idiosyncratic quality of the informant's responses. Group interviews can elucidate divergent perspectives for viewing the same situation, even by professionals with similar training and similar positions in the same institution. Group interviews were rarely planned in advance. They arose spontaneously out of the interview situation. Professional and participant bystanders would volunteer their answers to questions addressed to the designated respondent. This occurred frequently if I had gained access to physical areas provided for professional staff to congregate without being visible to the "public." In the emergency room at City Hospital, staff nurses, physician consultants, interns, residents, and attendants all gathered at the nurses' station. Interviews inside the nurses' station generally prompted wide participation.

Observation reduces the investigator's reliance on the actor's fallible memory and consciously or unconsciously distorted reports. Observing events similar to those described is a useful check on the validity and reliability of the informant's description. For example, in response to my question about aftercare, social worker 11 at City Hospital gave the following idealized response: "Doctors order home health care when appropriate." Observation on the medical ward staff meetings demonstrated that the physician's signature on the home health care application to welfare is a formality. The social worker decides how many days a week and how many hours of home health service the ex-patient is to have. In fact, one physician signed the form prepared by the social worker, and asked: "What does a homemaker do anyway?" (medical resident 5, CH).

Who can prescribe psychoactive medication? This is a very sensitive and controversial issue in the mental health profession. Legally, only physicians prescribe. Contemporary mental health ideology, however, emphasizes the equality and shared power of the psychiatrist, the psychiatric nurse, and the psychiatric social worker. A distinction between the authority or lack of authority to medicate is academically obscured. According to data gathered through interviewing, there was no confusion among professionals; only physicians prescribe medication. Subsequent observation, however, convinced me that the interview data were erroneous. On one occasion, psychiatric nurse 10 on a community visit to a nursing home "recommended" that an ex-patient be given Stellazine. The nursing home director administered the medication and dosage as recommended, and had the order countersigned by the house doctor. On another occasion in the City Hospital emergency room, the psychiatric nurse reported on a patient's behavior, and the following dialogue ensued:

> Psychiatrist 2: Give him 5 mg. Haldol.
> Psychiatric nurse 4: What about 2½? He's a small, thin man.
> Psychiatrist 2: Sure, whatever you say.

Observation occasionally uncovered facts concealed from the interviewer. For example, hospital placement organizations maintain confidential information identifying inferior nursing homes. Because placement staff fears political repercussions, blacklisting is a taboo topic. Information regarding the existence and use of such blacklists was never volunteered by professionals in interviews. I became aware of it while observing a Geriatric Specialist Team meeting. In response to my subsequent pointed questioning at different stations, professionals grudgingly acknowledged the blacklisting phenomenon.

A fundamental disadvantage of the observer approach is the difficulty in inferring reasons for behavior from the mere observation of behavior. When ascertaining the actors' perspective is a major purpose of the study, this is a serious problem. The use of interviews to supplement the observation was therefore essential. At times, the nature of the event being observed precluded any elaboration of the data through interviews. For example, when a nursing home "escapee," an attendant, and I made an appearance at the police station, the sergeant's overriding desire to clear the room made it perfectly clear that any further inquiry by the researcher would be out of order.

The Myth of the Unobtrusive Observer

Does the presence of an observer influence and therefore distort the behavior of those he observes? Since the same question can be raised with any measurement device used in the social sciences, the researcher's problem is one of minimizing and noting the effect. The methodology may distort the researcher's perceptions as well as the reality acted out by participants. Involvement in the field and direct experience with the data over a prolonged period produces a richness and depth of understanding, but it also obscures the investigator's objectivity.

Unless the researcher tries to camouflage his investigatory role completely and assume the part of a participant, his interview-observation behavior will rarely go unnoticed. The myth of the unobtrusive observer is perpetuated by social researchers who do not want to acknowledge their influence on their subjects. There are a very few exceptions, and they reflect unique situational circumstances. For example, while taking a break one afternoon in the Central State Hospital cafeteria, I had a chance to eavesdrop on two administrators who were discussing the state of the hospital.

Even in very informal environments where I conscientiously worked at keeping a low profile, there were reminders that my note taking had not been disregarded. In the senior citizen center, participants expected me to take notes as a demonstration of my true interest in their point of view. When center director 3 quietly asked me if I was getting the information I wanted, an elderly lady proudly intervened: "Well, he got a half a page of notes from me today!" (senior citizen 2). On another occasion at the senior citizen center, an elderly lady repeatedly advised me to put more milk in my coffee, then jokingly added: "You go ahead and take some more, then you can put that in your notes, how some old lady insisted that you put more milk in your coffee until you nearly ruined it." (senior citizen 3).

No matter how discreet you are, the mechanics of data recording become an event in the social world of the participants. As illustrated above, the effect is not necessarily disadvantageous to the researcher. This outcome is not unique to nonprofessional participants. Professionals respond similarly:

> Interviewer: Do you feel uneasy having someone around who writes down everything you say?
> Informant: Oh, no, I'm flattered! Besides it's fun giving away secrets of the institution. I feel so mischievous.

Whether or not it is desirable or advantageous, the presence of the observer modifies the definition of the social situation and alters the participants' behavior.

Events arise in which the supposedly unobtrusive observer must become an interventive actor. When I saw a confused elderly lady making her escape from the nursing home, I had two choices—to let her go and observe what happened or to intervene and see that she got back to the home before traveling too far. The former seemed unethical. My role as responsible citizen subverted my role as researcher. In another case, an elderly gentleman at Central State Hospital first assured himself of my confidentiality as an outsider and then proceeded to complain at great length about the conditions in the hospital. In fear of reprisal he did not take his complaints to the staff. When the staff team discussed his case, it concluded that he was "doing just fine, no complaints" and that there was "no need to rush." Even though I believed that his concealment of his complaints was a disservice to himself, I did not consider it my prerogative to tell the "real" story. I had been drawn into the situation because of my unique status on the service.

It should be remembered that the investigator enters the participants' world asking for cooperation, portraying himself as a friendly, congenial fellow. According to social conventions of reciprocity, participants sometimes ask the researcher to "return the favor." Most requests for advice or assistance can be conceded to or evaded without threatening the investigation. But the researcher is not always so fortunate. For example, one of my frequent informants on life inside the nursing home caught a midwinter cold. The nursing staff, according to the lady, had refused to give her aspirins without doctor's orders. When she asked me to buy her some, I felt the burden to "come through" or else discredit the illusion of friendship that I had cultivated. I smuggled in a small bottle of aspirin and made her promise to hide it and to refuse to divulge the name of her supplier if she were caught. I wanted to protect my good relations with the staff too.

REFERENCES

Anderson, Nancy. 1974. "Approaches to Improving the Quality of Long-Term Care for Older Persons." *The Gerontologist* 14 (December): 6.

Barnes, Jonathan A. 1974. "Effects of Reality Orientation Classroom on Memory Loss, Confusion, and Disorientation in Geriatric Patients." *The Gerontologist* 14 (April): 2.

Bauxbaum, Carl B. 1973. "Second Thoughts on Community Mental Health." *Social Work* 18. pp.25-29.

Becker, Howard. 1963. *Outsiders.* New York: The Free Press.

Butler, Robert N. 1974. "Life Review Therapy." *Geriatrics* (November).

——. 1973. *Aging and Mental Health: Positive Psycho-Social Approaches.* St. Louis: Mosley.

——. 1963. "The Life Review." *Psychiatry* 26: 65.

Cannicott, S. M. 1968. "Order Out of Confusion." *International Journal of Psychiatry.*

Caro, Francis G. 1975. "The Researcher-Practitioner Relationship." *Journal of Research and Development in Education.*

——. 1974. "Professional Roles in Maintenance of the Disabled Elderly in the Community: A Forecast." *The Gerontologist* 14 (August): 4.

——, ed. 1971. *Readings in Evaluation Research.* New York: Russell Sage Foundation.

Cartwright, R. S. 1968. "Psychotherapeutic Processes." In *Annual Review of Psychology,* ed. P. Farnsworth. Palo Alto: Annual Reviews.

Cohen, Ruth G. 1974. "Outreach and Advocacy in the Treatment of the Aged." *Social Casework* (May): 5.

Curtin, Sharon R. 1973. *Nobody Ever Died of Old Age.* Boston: Little, Brown, and Company.

Davis, Kingsley. 1938. "Mental Hygiene and Class Structure." *Psychiatry* 1.

Erikson, Kai T. 1962. "Notes on the Sociology of Deviance." *Social Problems* 9, pp.307-13.

——. 1961. *A Comparative Analysis of Complex Organizations.* New York: Free Press.

Fabricant, Michael. 1975. "Administering Juvenile Justice in an Urban Setting: Structure and Process in Perspective." Dissertation, Brandeis University.

Feigenbaum, E. M. 1974. "Geriatric Psychopathology, Internal or External?" *Journal of the American Geriatric Society* 22: 49.

Folsom, James, and Geneva Folsom. 1974. "The Real World." *Mental Hygiene* (Summer): 3.

Ford, D., and H. Urban. 1967. "Psychotherapy." In *Annual Review of Psychology,* ed. P. Farnsworth, p. 18. Palo Alto: Annual Reviews.

Gaitz, Charles. 1974. "Barriers to the Delivery of Psychiatric Services to the Elderly." *The Gerontologist* 14 (June): 3.

————, and Judith Scott. 1975. "Analysis of Letters to Dear Abby Concerning Old Age." *The Gerontologist* (February): 1.

Godbole, A., and U. Scott Verinis. 1974. "Brief Psychotherapy in the Treatment of Emotional Disorders in Physically Ill Geriatric Patients." *The Gerontologist* 14 (April): 2.

Goffman, Erving. 1961. *Asylums.* New York: Doubleday Anchor Books.

————. 1959. *The Presentation of Self in Everyday Life.* New York: Doubleday Anchor Books.

Goldfarb, Alvin. 1974. *Aging and Organic Brain Syndrome.* Fort Washington, Pa: McNeil Laboratories, monograph.

Goode, William J., and Paul Hatt. 1952. *Methods in Social Research.* New York: McGraw-Hill.

Gottesman, Leonard E., and Norman C. Bourestom. 1974. "Why Nursing Homes Do What They Do." *The Gerontologist* 14: 6.

Greenley, James, and Stuart Kirk. 1973. "Organizational Characteristics of Agencies and the Distribution of Services to Applicants." *Journal of Health and Social Behavior* 14 (March).

Hansen, Gary, Samuel Yoshioka, Marvin Taves, and Francis Caro. 1965. "Older People in the Midwest: Conditions and Attitudes." In *Old People and Their Social World,* ed. Arnold Rose and Warren Peterson. Philadelphia: Davis.

Harris, Raymond. 1975. "Breaking the Barriers to Better Health—Care Delivery for the Aged." *The Gerontologist* 15 (February): 1.

Hunt, R. C. 1958. "Ingredients of a Rehabilitation Program." In *An Approach to the Prevention of Disability from Chronic Psychosis. Proceedings of the 34th Annual Conference of the Milbank Memorial Fund, Part I, 1957.* New York: Milbank Memorial Fund.

Kaplan, Jerome. 1974. Editorial, "The Hospital Model: Curse or Blessing for Homes Serving the Aged." *The Gerontologist* 14 (August): 4.

Kirk, Stuart A., and James R. Greenley. 1974. "Denying or Delivering Services." *Social Work* (July).

Kitsuse, John I. 1962. "Societal Reaction to Deviant Behavior: Problems of Theory and Methods." *Social Problems* 9 (Winter): 247–57.

Kral, V. A. 1970. "Clinical Contributions Toward an Understanding of Memory Function." *Diseases of the Nervous System* 31.

Kramer, Morton, et al. 1971. "Patterns of Use of Psychiatric Facilities by the Aged: Past, Present, Future." Paper prepared for the National Institute of Mental Health, U.S. Department of Health, Education, and Welfare.

Lemert, Edwin. 1972. *Human Deviance, Social Problems, and Social Control*. Englewood Cliffs, NJ: Prentice-Hall.

————. 1951. *Social Pathology*. New York: McGraw-Hill.

Lieberman, Morton A. 1974. "Relocation Research and Social Policy." *The Gerontologist* 14 (December): 6.

Love, Edmund G. 1956. *Subways Are for Sleeping*. New York: Signet.

Lowenthal, Marjorie Fisk. 1967. *Aging and Mental Disorder in San Francisco*. San Francisco: Jossey-Boss.

Mann, John. 1971. "Technical and Social Difficulties in the Conduct of Evaluation Research." *Readings in Evaluation Research*, ed. Francis Caro. New York: Russell Sage Foundation.

Markson, Elizabeth W. 1974. "The Emperor's New Clothes—A Case Study of Instability on a Geriatric Service." *The Gerontologist* 14 (December): 6.

Markson, Elizabeth, Gary S. Levitz, and Maryvonne Gognalons-Caillard. et al. 1973. "The Elderly and the Community: Reidentifying Unmet Needs." *Journal of Gerontology* 28: 4.

Mayadas, Nazneer, and Douglas Hink. 1974. "Group Work with the Aging." *The Gerontologist* 14 (October): 5.

Meacher, Michael. 1972. *Taken for a Ride*. London: Longman.

Mechanic, David. 1969. *Mental Health and Social Policy*. Englewood Cliffs, N.J.: Prentice-Hall.

Mendelson, Mary A. 1974. *Tender Loving Greed*. New York: Knopf.

Mendelson, Mary. 1975. "In Her Own Words." *People* (March).

Miller, D. B. 1974. "Life Course of Patients Discharged from Two Nursing Homes." *The Gerontologist* 14 (October): 5.

Miller, E. 1968. "Psychological Theories of Electro-Convulsive Therapy." *International Journal of Psychiatry* 5.

Murrell, Stanley A. 1971. "An Open Systems Model for Psychotherapy Evaluation." *Community Mental Health Journal* 9 (Winter): 4.

Parsons, Talcott. 1949. *Essays on Sociological Theory, Pure and Applied*. Glencoe, Ill.: Free Press.

Patterson, Robert. 1971. *The Aged and Community Mental Health: A Guide to Program Development*, vol. 8, Report no. 81. New York: Group for the Advancement of Psychiatry.

Pfeiffer, Eric, and Ewald Busse. 1973. "Mental Disorders in Later Life—Affective Disorders; Paranoid, Neurotic, and Situational Reactions." In *Mental Illness in Later Life,* ed. Ewald Busse and Eric Pfeiffer. Washington, D.C.: American Psychiatric Association.

Pincus, A. 1970. "Reminiscence in Aging and Its Implication for Social Work Practice." *Social Work* 15: 47.

Redick, Richard, Morton Kramer, and Carl Taube. 1973. "Epidemiology of Mental Illness and Utilization of Psychiatric Facilities." In *Mental Illness in Later Life,* ed. Ewald Busse and Eric Pfeiffer. Washington, D.C.: American Psychiatric Association.

Rock, Ronald S., Marcus Jacobson and Richard Janopaul. 1968. *Hospitalization and Discharge of the Mentally Ill.* Chicago: University of Chicago Press.

Rosenhan, D. L. 1973. "On Being Sane in Insane Places." *Science,* January.

Rosow, Irving. 1962. "Old Age: One Moral Dilemma of an Affluent Society." *The Gerontologist* 2 (December): 4.

Saul, Sidney, and Sharon Saul. 1974. "Group Psychotherapy in a Proprietary Nursing Home." *The Gerontologist* 14 (October): 5.

Scheff, Thomas J. 1966. *Being Mentally Ill: A Sociological Theory.* Chicago: Aldine.

Scheff, Thomas J. 1964. "The Societal Reaction to Deviance: Ascriptive Elements in Psychiatric Screening of Mental Patients in a Midwestern State." *Social Problems* 11 (4) (Spring).

Schore, Herbert. 1974. "What's New About Alternatives." *The Gerontologist* 14 (February): 1.

Selltiz, Claire, Lawrence S. Wrightsman, and Stuart W. Cook. 1976. *Research Methods in Social Relations.* New York: Holt, Rinehart and Winston.

Simon, Alexander. 1973. "Mental Health and Mental Illness in Aging: An Overview." in *Community Mental Health and Aging: An Overview.* ed. Albert G. Feldman, Los Angeles: University of Southern California, Gerontological Center.

Schwartz, Morris S., and Charlotte G. Schwartz. 1964. *Social Approaches to Mental Patient Care.* New York: Columbia University Press.

Spitzer, Stephen, and Norman K. Denzin. 1968. *The Mental Patient: Studies in the Sociology of Deviance.* New York: McGraw-Hill.

Stannard, Charles I. 1973. "Old Folks and Dirty Work: The Social Conditions for Patient Abuse in Nursing Homes." *Social Problems* 20: 3.

Statistical Notes. Biometry Branch, Serial Publications. National Institute of Mental Health, U.S. Department of Health, Education, and Welfare. Washington, D.C.: Government Printing Office.

Stotsky, Bernard A. 1970. *The Nursing Home and the Aged Psychiatric Patient.* New York: Appleton Century Crofts.

Susser, Mervyn. 1968. *Community Psychiatry: Epidemiological and Social Themes.* New York: Random House.

Suster, Gerald. 1971. "A System of Groups in Institutions for the Aged." *Social Casework* (October): 8.

Thompson, William C., Jr. 1969. *Nursing Homes and Public Policy: Drift and Decision in New York State.* Ithaca: Cornell University Press.

Tobin, Sheldon. 1974. "How Nursing Homes Vary." *The Gerontologist* 14 (December): 6.

Toepfer, Caroline, et al. 1974. "Remotivation as Behavior Therapy." *The Gerontologist* (October): 5.

Wang, Shan W. 1973. "Special Diagnostic Procedures—The Evaluation of Brain Impairment." In *Mental Illness in Later Life,* ed. Ewald Busse and Eric Pfeiffer. Washington, D.C.: American Psychiatric Association.

Wasser, Edna. 1971. "Protective Practice in Serving the Mentally Impaired Aged." *Social Casework* 52 (October): 8.

Weinberg, George. 1970. *The Action Approach.* New York: New American Library.

Weinberg, Jack. 1974. "What Do I Say to My Mother When I Have Nothing to Say." *Geriatrics* (November).

————. 1957. "Psychotherapy of the Aged." In *Progress in Psychotherapy,* ed Masserman and Moreno, vol. 2. New York.

Whitehead, Anthony. 1970. *In the Service of Old Age: The Welfare of Psychogeriatric Patients.* Baltimore: Penguin.

Wilensky, Harold L., and Charles N. Lebeaux. 1965. *Industrial Society and Social Welfare.* New York: Free Press.

Wiseman, Jacqueline. 1970. *Stations of the Lost: The Treatment of Skid Row Alcoholics.* Englewood Cliffs, N.J.: Prentice-Hall.

ABOUT THE AUTHOR

DWIGHT FRANKFATHER is employed as a Research Associate in the Office of Program Planning and Research at the Community Service Society of Greater New York and is a part-time instructor at New York University. His special interest is the evaluation of service programs for the elderly.

Dr. Frankfather holds a B.A. from the University of Colorado and a Ph.D. from the Florence Heller School for Advanced Studies in Social Welfare at Brandeis University.

ALIENATION IN CONTEMPORARY SOCIETY: A Multidisciplinary Examination
edited by Roy S. Bryce-Laporte
Claudewell Thomas

COMMUNITY CONTROL OF HEALTH SERVICES: The Martin Luther King Health Center Community Management System
Noel M. Tichy

HOUSING THE ELDERLY
Elizabeth D. Huttman

PUBLIC POLICY TOWARD DISABILITY
Monroe Berkowitz
William G. Johnson
Edward H. Murphy

REGULATION AND EXPANSION OF HEALTH FACILITIES
Eleanore Rothenberg

RESETTLING RETARDED ADULTS IN A MANAGED COMMUNITY
Arnold Birenbaum
Samuel Seiffer

B1